Congratulations! W

competing, have a few shows under your belt, or are considered an "old pro" in this sport, this book was written for you!

Looking back at my first competition prep, I can now see that this book has literally been seven years in the making. Throughout those years I've experienced many "rookie" mistakes, learned invaluable information first hand from judges, located great resources that saved money and time, and so much more! The fire for this book was fueled even further as I ventured into selling competition suits. Upon coming into contact with numerous first time competitors, I noticed many of the girls had many questions, concerns, and situations regarding everything from how to choose a show, which categories to compete in, how to find a trainer, where to get shoes, what to expect the day of the competition, all the way to what to expect after it is all said and done. After answering these questions time and again I realized there was nothing offered, in one place, as a resource where all of these questions PLUS so many more could be answered. If I had a dime for every time I heard, "If only I had known..." well you know the rest.

Let's face it; this sport takes a lot of time, dedication, money, and willpower. Let me tell you, from experience, there is nothing worse than training for 6 months only to eat a steak, the night before the show, which has been soaked in sodium broth causing a 10 pound weight gain come stage time. I'm a firm believer in avoiding as many mistakes the first time out as possible, or more so, helping YOU avoid them without having to learn the hard way. Through my many years on stage, my experience as a judge, a lot of trial and error, and "rubbing elbows" with top judges and athletes in this industry it has become my number one goal to provide you with anything and everything related to competing. I've even included a Q and A section with top judges so you don't have to wonder what they are looking for, as well as a Q and A section with competitors representing different organizations and levels (amateurs and pro's) for further perspective, a professional photographer, and competitors who dealt with eating/body image disorders during competition prep.

So, it is with great excitement that I offer this book as the most comprehensive competition guide currently available to the female competitor. I have taken great care to cover the most frequently asked questions, to the not so frequently asked. I've enlisted the help of many top level competitors and judges who all share the same goal of making your competition experience as exciting and "mistake-free" as possible. I hope that this book will provide you with invaluable information no matter where you are at in your journey. With that being said, I wish you all "happy training" and may you all make, "First Call Out."

Chapter 1:

Choosing a Competition

You've made the decision to compete, so now what? Many first time competitors become a little overwhelmed when it comes time to choosing their first show. What organization should I compete in? Can I compete in multiple organizations? What is the difference between a tested and non-tested show? Where can I find a list of banned substances? Do I need to compete locally? Which category/categories should I enter? What is the difference between Bikini, Figure, Fitness, Women's Physique, and Bodybuilding? What does "cross- over" mean? Where can I find a listing of upcoming competitions? How many shows should I do? How much time do I need to get ready? Let's address each topic individually.

What organization should I compete in?

Choosing an organization is an important decision, as different ones have different requirements and stipulations. Let me break it down even further.

Tested vs Non-Tested: Some like to say "natural" vs.

"not natural," however I don't believe this is a fair or politically correct way to state it. Just because a show might be considered "not natural" doesn't mean that natural competitors (IE competitors not using any banned substances) aren't competing in this venue, therefore I prefer to label them as "tested" and "non-tested" shows.

A show that is "tested" means there are certain substances which you are not allowed to use if you want to participate in the competition, and a method of "testing" will be implemented (usually polygraph, urine, or both). Of course the main ones that immediately come to mind are steroids. However, there are NUMEROUS other substances that are not allowed, yet are readily found in over the counter supplements. Unfortunately, I have known girls who unknowingly take something banned because they bought it at their local supplement store, assuming it was "legal." It is not imperative to memorize the whole banned substance list, however it would be very wise to look at the list and compare the ingredients in your supplements to what is listed. If you have any questions regarding ingredients, DO NOT take it until you have contacted the promoter of the show to verify that it is allowed. You can find a list of banned substances at

http://www.thenaturalmusclenetwork.com/OCB/forms/DrugTestingGuidelines.pdf.

A non-tested show does not have any stipulations regarding what substances can be used. There isn't anything considered banned and no means of testing done. Let me just add, I have done many non-tested shows, while meeting all the requirements of a "natural" competitor and have won my categories, so don't let the stereotype of "non- tested" detour you from considering the show.

Once you have decided between tested and non-tested, it's time to consider where organization will best match your decision.

NANBF: The NANBF (nanbf.org), the North American Natural Bodybuilding Federation, is one of the main amateur natural bodybuilding organizations. The professional Federation associated with the NANB is called the IFPA (http://www.thenaturalmusclenetwork.com/IFPA/index.htm). Usually to attain professional status you must win the overall in your category. I will discuss what is meant by "overall" later in the book. This is just a basic "rule of thumb" however; I have seen Pro status awarded to everyone who is competing for overall. It is up to the discretion of the Federation and can change from show to show. As a side note, let me add that when you are looking at the information regarding a show, you will want to take note that the show is indeed labeled as a "Pro Qualifier." There will also be details as to which categories are eligible for Professional status. As with any questions, if you are unsure about anything, you should contact the show promoter for clarification.

NPC: The NPC (npcnewsonline.com), National Physique Committee, is the main amateur "Non-tested" organization. The professional federation associated with the NPC is called the IFBB. Attaining professional status through the IFBB is different than that of the NANBF. As with the NANB you must first make sure that the NPC show you are considering is labeled as a "National Qualifier." Again, the categories which are considered for National qualification will be stated on the entry form or the show site. Usually, but sometimes with exception, the top three placements in the category are eligible to compete in a National level show. Each National show has different criteria for who will receive IFBB status. Some shows give IFBB status to Overall winners only. Some will award it to the top two in each class, and some will award it to the top three Overall winners. Again, each promoter and show clearly states who will be eligible for IFBB status. If you have questions or concern contact the show promoter. As a final note, the NPC does offer "tested" shows as well. These shows will clearly state "tested" on the show information sheet.

WBFF: The WBFF (wbffshows.com),World Bodybuilding and Fitness Federation, is a relatively new amateur organization, although it seems to be growing by leaps and bounds. I admittedly do not know much about this organization although I do have quite a few friends who compete in the WBFF and absolutely love it. From what I do gather, it is more of a "production" where they highly emphasize putting on a show for the competitors as well as the spectators. The most highly noted difference between the WBFF and other organizations is the categories that are offered to compete in, including a theme wear and evening gown division. They also offer an opportunity to receive Professional status. The means in which to attain this, as well as everything there is to know about the organization can be found on their site. I copied their Mission Statement from their site to give you an idea of what they are founded on.

The desired public image of our company is to give athletes a venue in which they can compete, and be treated with the utmost professionalism. The key strategic influence is to promote health and fitness in a rapidly growing industry. Our target market is a health and fitness conscious individual who wants to embark on or develop a professional career within the health and fitness industry. Ultimately the WBFF seeks to raise a standard in bodybuilding, fitness, and modeling, and give athletes an unlimited opportunity. Our expectations are to promote our company, our athletes, and our sponsors to the best of our ability while becoming internationally known as a reputable and conscientious corporation.

Before moving on, let me also add that there are other organizations/federations as well such as the OCB, AFPA, WNBF and many others. I introduced the above mentioned due to the fact they are the largest among the groups. Almost all federations and their corresponding shows can be found at www.bodybuilding.com under "contests." They all will state whether they are a tested or non-tested show as well as the stipulations required to move on to pro status within that organization.

Where can I find a list of competitions?

Each of the organizations has a list of upcoming competitions on their site. You should refer to the corresponding links provided above to see the schedule. It is important to note that sometimes available shows are NOT listed on the site. Another resource available to find upcoming events can be found at www.bodybuilding.com under "contests" (located on left hand side of site).

Usually fitness oriented places of business like a gym or supplement store will have fliers advertising local competitions hanging up. Almost all gyms have at least one person who is involved in the competition circuit and would be a great resource in finding out information regarding any upcoming shows.

Should I compete locally or consider a show out of state?

One thing to consider when deciding on a show is the location of the venue. A local show is generally considered one you don't have to travel or book a hotel for. I use the word "generally" due to the fact that even though it might not be necessary to stay in a hotel for a show you can easily attend, some competitors choose to stay in the host hotel out of convenience and easy access to the venue.

Almost all promoters take the time in securing a "host hotel" in order to accommodate competitors. The hotel usually sets a number of rooms aside at a discounted rate specifically for people participating in the show. The hotel contact information, including phone number and address are almost always provided on the competition entry form. I will get into further detail regarding an out of town show in a later chapter.

Many competitors prefer a local show for their first competition experience for convenience as well as cutting down on traveling expenses. The choice regarding local vs. out of town is completely up to you.

How many shows can I compete in?

There really is no set answer to this. If this is your first show and you are not sure if you will want to compete in the future, your best bet is to pick one show and see how you feel about participating in another one afterwards. Some girls just know they are only interested in getting through one and don't even consider multiple competitions. Others go into as "testing the waters," so to speak, and decide what action they want to take once they've made it through their first one. I've also seen girls very excited and gung ho about doing as many shows as they can, only to get through the first one and realize one was plenty. I've also seen the opposite; a new competitor who only had the intention of doing one show had such a great experience they immediately look for another one to compete in. You won't know how you feel about competing until you go through the whole process of preparation and the competition itself.

Can I compete in different Federations/Organizations?

The quick answer is yes. If you compete in the NANBF one weekend and decide you want to compete in a NPC show the next weekend, there is no rule against it. In fact, I would highly recommend considering competing in a couple different organizations as it gives you a point of reference in deciding which path you would like to take. The only time it could be questionable to compete in multiple federations is when you obtain professional status. Some professional federations have stipulations regarding this topic. I've seen some "allow" the cross over as long as you have not placed top three in a pro show, some don't allow their pro's to compete in other organizations at all, and some don't have any rules regarding this. On the amateur level it is never an issue (unless one comes up sometime between now and the time this book is published), but again, you should always make sure you are knowledgeable of the different rules regarding each level of competitor status.

Which category should I enter?

There really is no easy answer for this question, although it is probably the most important thing to consider when entering your first competition. As of right now, the categories for female competitors are: Bikini, Figure, Fitness, Women's Physique, and Bodybuilding. Why do I say, "As of right now"? This sport is growing by leaps and bounds and is changing constantly. As a point of reference, when I entered my first competition seven years ago, the categories to choose from were: Figure, Fitness, and Bodybuilding. It wasn't until my third year that Bikini was introduced and I specifically remember there being four competitors in that category. Fast forward to now…Bikini is now the largest category for female competitors. As far as Women's Physique is concerned, this category has only been around for about two years and is growing at an exponentially fast rate. So, is it possible for another category to have come or gone as you are reading this? Absolutely!! But for now, we will stick to these five categories.

Knowing which category you should enter basically comes down to your body composition. For example, a woman competing in the Bikini division looks very different from a Bodybuilder. In fact, if you have the physical make up of a bodybuilder and enter yourself in the Bikini division, you should brace yourself as you will not fare well in the placements and can be pretty much guaranteed all judges' comments will say the same thing, "You are in the wrong category and should be competing as a bodybuilder." This is a very drastic scenario and given for the sake of making a point. However, sometimes it really does get tricky in choosing which one to enter. The criteria for Women's Physique are summed up as "A big Figure competitor." How's that for clarification? Are you more suited for Figure or do you have just a tad too much muscle and need to move up to Physique? This is a very gray area for sure. If you don't have a trainer or outside source to help you find your placement, sometimes you have to just pick one or both categories and see where the judges place you. Consider it trial and error.

It is also possible to fit into one category one year and have to switch to a different one the next. When I first competed, I entered Figure every time. Of course my decision was easy due to the fact Physique didn't even exist. However, over the years of training and due to putting on a significant amount of muscle (and the introduction of Physique) the class I "fit" into best became a bit confusing. I asked friends who were knowledgeable about the criteria for the different categories which I should enter. Unfortunately everyone was "torn" on what I should do. To some I looked more like a "bigger Figure" and to others I was a "smaller Physique" competitor. The advice I was given was to enter both categories and let the judges decide. Again, if you are unsure of where you TRULY fit in, your best bet is to enter the categories you are torn between and let the judges choose for you.

So what IS the difference between categories?

The MAIN differences between categories usually come down to two things: muscle mass and body fat. Listed from least amount of muscle mass to the most: Bikini, Figure, Fitness (most resembles a Figure competitor in structure, but performs a gymnastic/tumbling routine as part of their judging criteria), Women's Physique, and Bodybuilding. (Currently the NANBF does not have a Women's Physique category)

It is important to familiarize yourself with the predominant characteristics and judging criteria of each category. More in-depth information regarding posing and presentation will be discussed in a later chapter. Here is the judging criterion the NPC has set forth regarding each category (All this information can be found on their site):

Bikini:

Judges will be scoring competitors using the following criteria:

- Balance and Shape
- Overall physical appearance including complexion, skin tone, poise and overall presentation.

Figure:

Scoring – Judges will be scoring competitors using the following criteria:

- Small degree of muscularity with separation, no visible striations
- Overall muscle tone with shapely lines, overall firmness and not excessively lean

- Full general assessment
- Healthy appearance
- Make-up
- Skin tone

Fitness:

Judges will score the degree of athleticism using the following criteria:

- Firmness
- Symmetry
- Proportion
- Overall physical appearance including –
  1. Complexion
  2. Poise
  3. Overall Presentation

Scoring – Round 2:

Judges will use four (4) aspects to score this round using the following criteria:

1. Strength – the amount and types of strength moves.

   A. The degree of difficulty of these moves.

   B. The ease and correctness of the moves

1. Flexibility – the number and types of flexibility moves

A. The degree of difficulty of these moves

B. the ease and correctness of the moves

1. Cardiovascular – the tempo of the routine

2. Overall Package – Full general assessment including but not limited to creativity, stage presence, outfits, hair and make-up

Women's Physique:

JUDGING CRITERIA

* Symmetry, shape, proportion, muscle tone, poise and beauty flow

* Physique assessment and comparison will take place during prejudging

Women's Physique Division has been created to give a platform for women, who enjoy weight training, competing, contest preparation. Competitors should display a toned, athletic physique showcasing femininity, muscle tone, beauty/flow of physique.

The following are examples of common terms used in the bodybuilding industry. These words can be helpful to assess what should **not** be descriptive to the physiques being judged in women's physique:

Ripped, shredded, peeled, striated, dry, diced, hard, vascular, grainy, massive, thick, dense, etc.

While all types of physiques will be considered when it comes to height, weight, structure, etc. Excessive muscularity should be scored down accordingly.

Women's physique competitors should have the overall aesthetics and look that is found in figure with a little more overall muscularity.

Bodybuilding:

Judges will score competitors according to the NPC "total package" which is a balance of size, symmetry and muscularity.

How much time do I need to get ready for my competition?

Another important factor in choosing a show is how long it gives you to prepare. There is no set time regarding this and is highly dependent on your current body composition. Obviously the more change you need to accomplish is going to require a longer amount of time. There does seem to be a "standard" amount of time taken that ranges between twelve and sixteen weeks, however all factors including current muscle mass and body fat need to be considered. For my first show, I allowed six months to prepare but now only require approximately four months. The good news is that prepping for subsequent competitions usually, but not always, takes less time as you are not starting from scratch.

Now that you've (hopefully) chosen a competition and (hopefully) know which category to enter, it's time to start your preparation for the big day! So, what now?

Chapter 2
Competition Prep-Part 1

If you have never gone through competition prep, the next logical question you probably have is, "So what exactly do I need to do to get ready?" The answer to this is: diet, train, pose, sleep, repeat.

Diet:

You've heard the saying, "Abs are made in the kitchen." If this statement has ever proven to be true, it is found in competition prep. The nutrition plan you follow will be one of the key factors in determining your success come show time. When you tell people, who are not familiar with the competition preparation process, you are dieting they will assume you are following a popular weight loss diet and are on a quest to drop a few pounds. If you share this belief, you are about to be in for a huge surprise. It is safe to say that the diet is among the top reason why people decide NOT to compete. It is not for the faint of heart, but the payoff and gratification you will feel is well worth it. If I haven't scared you off, let's continue on.

If you have no clue as to how to go about picking a nutrition and/or workout plan, it is imperative that you find someone who DOES know how to get you where you need to be. Let's look at your options.

Online:

With the vast online resources available today, you can simply go to a search engine and type in, "nutrition plan for competition" and receive a plethora of choices. Many competitors have willingly shared their nutrition program via articles and personal websites for free. Even fitness/bodybuilding magazines feature articles showcasing competitors and the nutrition/workout regimen they followed. Although this method is definitely considered the cheapest route to go, it is also the most flawed. You must be aware that the plan they followed was designed for them. Just because they consumed carbohydrates with every meal doesn't mean YOUR body can reach competition level following the same plan. It is also a safe bet that the plan represented was only followed at a specific time, therefore does not reflect any changes made as time/progress went on. Most nutrition plans are changed or altered a few times, depending on how close the competition date is and how your body is reacting. It never hurts to look at these plans to get an idea of what to expect, however, I would consider other resources first.

Friends:

Friends who compete can be a great source of information. If you know someone who would be willing to share their nutrition plan with you then you might enlist their help. Without sounding unappreciative of well-meaning friends, it is important to be aware of their "success" with regards to competing. If they did not place well and their number one critique was they needed to be leaner, then following the same diet might not be the best idea. However, if they did do very well, this could still be a viable option. One thing to keep in mind, as stated in the online resource, is the diet you are going to follow was designed for THEM and not for YOU. Just because your friend had great success with the plan does not guarantee you will also. If they have been involved with the competition world for a few years, are knowledgeable about numerous nutrition plans, and are confident they can provide you with a custom nutrition plan then this could be an excellent option with little to no cost.

Spouse/Significant Other

Having a spouse or significant other (SO for short) can also be a viable choice if they have experience with competition training. There are some great benefits enlisting their help, include getting your plan for free, constant/daily monitoring of your progress, and immediate advice or answers to any questions or concerns that come up. It can also be a great tool to ensure you stay on track and are not tempted to go off plan. The water retention and/or bloat caused by a cheat meal is harder to hide from someone who sees your body on a daily basis.

Let me offer a word of caution when considering this option. You must establish clear cut rules, expectations, and guidelines from the beginning. Speaking from experience, since my husband trained me for some of my shows, it is very easy to blur the line between trainer and spouse. On a few occasions I was known to approach my husband with the puppy dog eyes stating how hungry I was for hot wings and pizza and felt like I "deserved" the cheat due to my quick progress. He would say, "As your husband I want you to be happy, but as your trainer I don't think you should." Or if on the other hand he would say, "You can have a cheat meal" I would say, "Are you sure? If I'm not lean enough I'm blaming you!"

You also need to be open to receiving criticism. If your SO suggests it is time to make further dietary changes or increase cardio it is not wise to say, "What? Are you calling me fat?" If you feel it could be difficult to separate the professional part of your relationship from the private, skipping this option is probably your best bet. However, if you are willing to treat the situation as if someone else was training you and can talk about what you expect from each other on this level, this could be a great choice.

Trainer:

Hiring a trainer for the sole purpose of helping you prepare for a competition is probably the most effective way to ensure your success. With that being said, it is probably the most expensive option as well. Do not underestimate the accountability factor of a trainer. If you are on the fence about eating that piece of pizza or not, the sheer knowledge that your trainer will see you in a suit the next day could be all the convincing you need to go ahead with the scheduled egg whites. If your nutrition plan is among the highest factor in determining your success, it goes without saying that finding the right trainer goes hand in hand with this.

Finding the right trainer can seem a little overwhelming, but it doesn't have to be. I don't want to be passé in this regard, but it can be as simple as asking around. The world of bodybuilding (I'm grouping all categories into one for simplification sake) is a very tight knit community. This will become apparent to you as you start competing in multiple local shows and notice many of the same people showing up to each one. This is of great benefit when looking for a trainer because word of mouth, either good or bad, spreads like wildfire within the competition community. If you see someone at your gym who looks like they compete, it's as easy as asking them who their trainer is. Usually they will be more than happy to provide that information. If you see a trainer in the gym that looks like they compete, you can ask them if they train competitors and request some references.

Once you locate a potential trainer, the next thing you need to do is make sure this is going to be a good "fit" for you. Trainers, after all, are human and come with different personalities and philosophies regarding nutrition/training. Let's discuss some important topics regarding choosing a trainer (in no particular order):

Qualifications:

Although I stated these were in no particular order, the trainer's qualifications are probably the most important thing to consider. I'm going to break it down even further:

Have they trained past competitors?

Although it isn't a MUST, it is definitely strongly encouraged to find someone who is familiar with training FEMALES for a competition. I'm not being sexist or discriminatory but let's face it, a female has hormones and other issues a male does not have. If a trainer has only successfully trained men, it is plausible he isn't fully aware of how a nutrition plan needs to differ between a male and female. I know plenty of male trainers who are highly successful in training females, so be open to a male trainer...just make sure they have experience with female competitors.

How did well did their clients do in the competition?

Don't be afraid to ask the trainer to see pictures of female competitors they have helped. If they have confidence in their ability to train you, they will have no problem offering up pictures and/or names and contact information for people they have worked with.

Although it's definitely a good attribute to have successful competitors, you must keep in mind that a trainer is only as good as the client. In other words, you must remember that a trainer is a tool in helping you achieve success and things like genetics and dedication need to be factored in. The trainer could be extremely qualified, but if the person following the plan constantly strays from the plan they are given then it is not the fault of the trainer. Same can be said for genetics. A trainer can only do so much with what he/she is given to work with. Just because a girl has decided to compete, doesn't mean she is genetically gifted or is built to do well in a competition. So, although the success of past clients is important, it is not a sole determinant in picking a trainer.

How long have they been training competitors?

This is important although not crucial. Everyone has to start at some point. Even the highly sought after trainer to the Pro's at one time had only a few months' worth of experience. If a trainer has only trained five competitors but they all won their show, then I think it would be wise to keep them as a potential trainer.

Do they compete?

A benefit to working with someone who has competed is that they have been through everything you are about to go through and therefore can offer advice and support along the way. They know what is required and expected of a competitor and will have other resources for you regarding other odds and ends of competing. Is it necessary to hire someone who has competed? I guess not. However, you are probably doing yourself a huge injustice by not working with someone who has gone through it.

How long have they been competing?

This is another qualification that is good to know, but not a deal breaker. Just stands to reason that someone who has been competing for a couple months might not be as knowledgeable as someone who has competed for ten years. If I had written this book after one year of competing, it would be significantly different than it is now. Time equals experience.

Cost:

Trainers are not cheap, especially the ones who have become well known for providing excellent services. They are among the top when it comes to the expenses you will incur on your journey to the stage. Many trainers have their cost broken down into different program options you can choose from. Some of these are based on a time period (IE a 12 week period), some are dependent on if you want personal training sessions, some are made up of nutrition/workout plans only, and others offer a flat competition rate plan. Again, if you are going to a trainer who is well known and sought after you can expect to put out a significant amount of money.

There are some Professional competitors who also offer training via online. This usually includes all correspondence being done via emails, pictures, and possibly phone calls. You can expect to receive a nutrition and workout plan which will be periodically changed throughout your prep. Most if not all of your progress will be determined by sending him/her pictures of yourself in different poses at scheduled times. Professional competitors, especially very well-known ones, are very busy and realize their time and knowledge are very valuable thus charge accordingly. As a point of reference, a friend of mine hired a very successful professional body builder for a 12 week plan and paid $2000 for the service. This should be considered an accurate estimate in what to expect if you go this route.

Payments:

If you don't have a significant amount of extra money lying around, then it would be beneficial to find out if the trainer accepts payments. Most trainers are aware of this and do offer payment plans. The only thing to take note of here is any "refund" policy. Be sure to ask about refunds or payments still owed if something should happen and you change your mind regarding competition. The safest assumption is no refunds will be given and all monies will still be expected in full.

Personality:

You can usually figure out someone's personality within the first couple minutes upon meeting. If at any time you feel uncomfortable or feel intimidated by a potential trainer, consider continuing your search. Some people want a "drill sergeant" and some prefer a more casual or personal approach.

There are going to be times during your prep where your emotions are going to take over, concerns will arise, and personal problems might need addressed. If you don't feel comfortable talking to your trainer about these issues, or they don't have the personality/compassion required to deal with your problems, it could be a long and lonely prep for you. Keep in mind your trainer is just that…your trainer. They are not there to be your therapist; however, as an example if you lose your period (which is common and discussed later) you need to be comfortable approaching this subject with him/her. Don't forget the fact you will most likely be standing half dressed in a posing suit in front of this person at some point in your training. Being comfortable with your trainer should be a high priority.

Philosophy:

Different people have different philosophies regarding certain topics. It is important to be "on the same page" so to speak with your trainer regarding some important topics. Here are some of the main ones to discuss:

Diet:

There is not one set way to achieving a competition ready physique. In fact, I have personally tried three different nutrition plans throughout my competition history and have had great success with each. What was the deciding factor on which one to follow? It all came down to choosing the plan I felt would be the "easiest" for me to stick to.

Some trainers believe in low carbs plans, some follow a high carb in the morning/low in the evening plan, and some implement a rotation. Protein needs are pretty much universal among trainers, but even that amount depends on your current body composition and the goal you are trying to achieve. Your fat intake can also vary significantly between trainers with different nutritional beliefs.

Chances are you have somewhat of an idea of how your body responds to different foods. If after sharing your knowledge, your trainer is still set on doing it his/her way and you are not comfortable with the plan you can either give their plan a try or seek out someone who shares similar dietary beliefs as you do. Remember, you will be following this nutritional format for at least 12 weeks, if you can't stand the thought of eating chicken but your trainer insists, you could be in for a long and miserable journey.

With that being said, don't expect to find a reputable trainer who is willing to let you have bacon wrapped sirloin with a loaded baked potato on a regular basis, if at all. Remember, the nutrition plan to prep for a show is what makes and breaks people from ever making it to the stage. I've personally seen people back out four weeks from a show they have dieted for diligently for eight weeks because they just couldn't stand doing the diet for even one more day. The road to the stage is not for the faint of heart, so don't make it harder on yourself by forcing yourself to follow a diet that consists mainly of food you can't stand to eat. A good trainer will take your taste preferences into consideration when designing a plan.

Workouts:

If you haven't guessed it yet, you can expect to spend a good amount of time at the gym. Don't be surprised when you feel as if the gym has become your second home. We will discuss what to look for in a gym in the next chapter.

The reason it is important to know the trainer's philosophy regarding training is really just to prepare yourself for what you should expect. Some trainers (like my husband) believe that if your diet is a perfect match for you then cardio should be kept at a bare minimum to avoid burning muscle or causing injury from so much wear and tear. Some trainers believe in doing cardio for a short time on an empty stomach first thing in the morning. Some follow a high intensity routine, while others suggest doing a morning and an evening session. Basically your cardio session(s) can be as little as NONE to as much as two hours a day. Best to find out what you can expect ahead of time so it doesn't come as a surprise. Of course your body fat percentage and how long until show time will be huge considerations in determining how much cardio is needed and could change throughout the process.

Personal Training:

If you are familiar with weight training and the exercises your trainer wants you to perform, there really is no need to be trained one-on-one on a consistent basis. However, there are advantages of personal training sessions. A personal training session with a trainer can ensure you are keeping correct form, lifting adequate weight, and pushing yourself above and beyond. Let's face it, when lifting the weight starts to hurt, most of us set it down no matter what repetition we might be on. If a trainer expects you to perform the movement 15 times and you are tempted to put it down on rep number 10, chances are a trainer will push you further than you would have pushed yourself had you been working out alone. Again, this is not necessary, but could be of benefit to you.

Supplements:

I know this is a hot topic, but it is also a very important one which needs to be addressed. I specifically want to address the use of steroids or other banned substances. Yes, I said the "S" word. I'm certain that anyone reading this is well aware of the use of banned substances in the world of bodybuilding. I make no judgments, either for or against them, and believe this is a personal decision that should be left up to the one making the choice. This is not brought up as a platform for debate, merely to emphasize the importance in making sure your trainer supports YOUR beliefs and desires regarding their use.

Your beliefs and feelings regarding this subject are very important when choosing a trainer and should be candidly talked about between the two of you. If you are competing in a tested show, and the trainer across from you obviously wouldn't qualify for a tested show, it is important to establish that he/she is willing to keep you natural and won't be constantly pushing anything on you. I've never come across any trainer who is forceful in this matter, but some have offered up the suggestion along the way. If they are clear as to your beliefs and goals, they should support your decision and be willing to take you on as a client.

On the flipside, if you are considering taking anything considered banned, it is just as important to make sure you are dealing with someone who is very knowledgeable in this matter. Almost all supplements have side effects and affect the body in different ways. Just as with any medicine or prescription, all supplements and dosage are dependent on many factors; it is of upmost importance to make sure you are dealing with someone who knows everything there is to know regarding the considered supplement. It would be just as unwise to seek the help of a trainer who only trains clients for tested shows if you are planning on using additional supplements.

Again, I know this is a hush-hush topic, but it is an important one. Either route you decide on just make sure you are informed and are in agreement with any potential trainer.

Who are they doing this for?

This topic wouldn't really have been discussed even as soon as about a month prior to writing this book, however, I have realized this can also be a point to consider. A friend of mine, after stepping off stage, got "cornered" by her trainer and was immediately reprimanded for everything from her posing to her appearance. This in itself was devastating to her, but the final straw was when her trainer said, "This isn't about YOU, this is about ME and my reputation."

Hopefully you understand this is absolutely not true and not acceptable. A trainer is a tool in helping you achieve your goals, and the whole process is 100% ONLY about you. If a trainer is more concerned about how you are going to further their business or overly focused on how your placement is going to affect them, take heed and look for someone else. Unfortunately, there are a few trainers who have built their reputation by heavily doting and advertising the "winners" they train. This is great if you are among one of them and share the same goal, however, if you are doing this for other reasons than just winning this could be a conflict. Also consider if a trainer does not believe you will benefit their reputation, they might not be willing to give you as much attention and guidance as a "star" competitor.

Again, I would have never thought this topic even a possibility if I had not seen a friend and fellow competitor go through this just recently. I am confident that most trainers realize this is about YOU and YOUR goals; just be cautious.

Final note:

These are just some of the main points, questions, and things to consider when looking for a trainer that is right for you. It would be wise to sit down prior to the first meeting and write down all topics you want to discuss. Remember, you are basically interviewing them for a job, and an important one at that! Don't be concerned about being upfront and honest about any and all topics you feel are important.

Also, if for some reason during training you realize he/she is not what you had expected, do not hesitate looking for a different person to help you. You might lose any money that was paid, but your success, happiness, and confidence in your trainer should outweigh anything else.

Chapter 3

Competition Prep-Part 2

I divided the competition prep into two parts as I believe they are both so fundamentally important, each deserve their own chapter. Your nutrition and training are the two key elements in your preparation. Sleep is just as important, and will be discussed later.

Now that you have chosen a trainer, he/she will most certainly give you the diet and workout plan they would like for you to follow. Because your diet has been created specifically for you, not much more discussion can go into the topic except to once again stress the importance of adhering to the plan you have been given.

This brings us to the topic of training. If you are currently a member of a gym, you might need to reassess its amenities to make sure it now accommodates your new goal as a competitor. If you do not currently belong to a gym, you now have the mission of choosing your "home away from home." Just as it was important to find the right trainer, the right gym is a main consideration to ensure success.

Location:

Right now the cost of gas is approximately $3.70 a gallon here in the Midwest and I'm certain those on the Coast are paying even more. Considering you will be going to the gym approximately six days a week; sometimes twice a day, the location of the gym is one of high importance. There might be a brand new facility 40 miles from your home that is all the rave, but do you REALLY want to be making that haul at 4:00am just to turn around go back again for a later cardio session at 6:00pm? Even if you have a fuel efficient car that gets 40 miles to the gallon, you will have to figure based on a six day a week workout, twice a day back and forth, spending about $60 a week just in trips to and from the gym. Draw that out over a month and you practically have another car payment.

Those of you who live in a rural area might be at the mercy of whatever facility is available, but for those of you who live in the city or within the vicinity, you should have a least a couple options to choose from.

As like with other topics, your best bet could be to talk with someone who also competes and find out where they train, if they like it, cost etc. If you don't happen to know anyone who could help you in this regard, then the next best thing to do is look around your immediate area for gyms nearby.

Once you locate a few possibilities, here are a few things you should consider before you make your final decision:

Cost:

If I haven't made it well known yet, the cost of competing in this sport is not cheap. There will seem a time when you are putting money out left and right for things you haven't had to deal with at this point (nails, hair, tanning, entry fees etc.). So, unless you have a fairly decent disposable income, the cost of your gym membership will most likely be one of your top concerns.

I don't know if it is considered brash or not, but when I walk into a facility the first thing I ask is, "How much are the monthly dues?" Usually most sales people are trained to show you around and tell you how wonderful the place is and leave the cost for the very end of the tour. The hope is you will be so enamored with the facility you will start to rationalize the monthly cost, even if your first instinct is that it is outside your budget. If it IS outside your comfort zone, simply thank them for their time and tell them you are just checking around for rates. Of course, you can save the leg time by calling ahead and asking for rates over the phone.

Hours:

Do you work full time? Are you going to have to work out really early before work, or later in the evening after you feed the family dinner? The hours of operation are crucial to your success. If you need to train at 4:00am in order to have adequate time to complete your workout before work, it won't do you any good to join a gym that doesn't open until 5:00am.

The facilities that now operate 24/7 are increasing in number. In fact, there are two facilities within a 5 mile radius of my home that offer this service. One of them actually has someone at the front desk at all times, and the other provides you with an electronic key which can be scanned to unlock the front door. These can be your absolute best bet if you can only workout at odd or inconsistent hours. Another benefit is their availability even during a holiday.

Daycare:

If you have any kids and will require the use of a daycare, this is a very important detail to consider. If they do provide daycare services, you will need to make sure the hours of availability will coincide with the time you will be working out. Most gyms consider the daycare an extra fee, so make sure this is considered into your monthly cost when considering the facility.

Contracts:

Gyms have come a long way in the past few years by offering monthly contracts. It has become standard practice for most facilities to offer the month to month memberships which gets you out of having to commit to one place for a full year. The payment plans can vary from place to place so make sure and inquire about each option they provide. Sometimes a significant discount is given by purchasing a longer period of time upfront. Another option, sometimes provided, is the ability to freeze your membership for a limited amount of time (usually two or three months) without having to pay. This can be useful, especially after your competition, when you aren't so inclined to hit the gym on a regular basis. (More on this later)

How busy is the facility? :

To some, this might not seem like anything of much importance. However, let me caution you about how difficult it will be to train and accomplish what you have set out to do, if the gym is always busy and you cannot get access to the pieces of equipment you need. If you know you will be working out at 6:00pm, you will be doing yourself a huge favor by asking the sales person approximately how many people workout around that time. If he/she says, "That's our busiest time, this place is pretty much packed!" then that needs to be a consideration. This isn't a deal breaker by any means, but once you've stood around waiting a few times for someone to get off of the piece of equipment you need, it gets old real fast.

Other competitors:

While on the subject of the number of members, you should also find out of there is anyone else who competes and trains out of their facility. If another competitor (or two or three…) use the gym to train for their shows, it is a good chance the facility is adequately equipped for your show prep. Plus, as stated before, it is always nice to have access to other competitors' knowledge and advice. Of course this is not a make or break option in your consideration, but is certainly a bonus.

Equipment:

Usually the larger, well established gyms have more to offer in this department. However, this is not a set in stone standard and some smaller gyms provide everything you will need. The gym I train at is smaller in comparison to some, and brand new, however it was opened by people who compete or do some serious weight lifting. Therefore, every piece of equipment in the facility purchased was well thought out in order to provide every exercise I could possibly do.

As a side note here, make sure and locate the dumb bells and note how heavy they go. Without making it sound sexist, usually this is a bigger concern for the male competitors. I do have a couple female bodybuilder friends who can out lift many of the guys in the gym, so I know this is an important factor. If you can throw around 110 pound weights like it's nothing, then it is important to have dumb bells that accommodate you. If the maximum weight goes up to 70 pounds, you are going to have to figure something out one way or another.

The two main equipment considerations can be broken down into weights and cardio. If the place is loaded with plenty of dumb bells, free weights, and a large variety of weight training equipment that offers a variety of exercises that can be performed, you are in business. However, if you see one squat rack and one leg extension machine as the extent of the pieces offered for a leg workout, this could be a red flag. The best case scenario would be you are the only one working legs on that given day. The worst case (and most likely) you will be doing a lot of walking lunges or won't be working legs at all.

Cardio equipment should not be overlooked either. If you are on a training program that requires you to spend a good amount of time doing cardiovascular exercise, you will appreciate a nice piece of equipment. The machines at the gym I train at are all equipped with a monitor that provides cable TV, IPod connection, and different graphics/tracks I can look at while exercising. Of course this is not a must have, but during one competition prep, I was doing 1.5 hours of cardio a day, 6 days a week, so it was definitely a nice distraction to have those options.

Besides the quality of equipment, take note of how many pieces are available as well as the variety provided. There are numerous methods of achieving your cardio workout including, but not limited to: treadmill, elliptical machine, recumbent bike, upright bike, stair mill (escalator), and stair stepper. Having a variety of machines to choose from can definitely help break up the monotony from day to day. Having access to a large amount of equipment can ensure there will be a piece available for you to use when you are ready.

Atmosphere:

As you are taking the tour of the facility, take note of the overall atmosphere of the gym. Do you feel it is conducive to your goals? Will you feel comfortable training there? Remember, you will be spending a lot of time there, so it is important to find a place you will actually enjoy being in.

I'm not saying anything negative against the YMCA, but that facility works well in making my point clear regarding different atmospheres. Obviously, there is a very wide variety of people who work out at the YMCA and range from very young (they let kids as young as 10 use the equipment) to the elderly. I have been a member of the YMCA during one of my comp prep's and actually had to wait on a young kid to get off the equipment I needed. I've also been involved in conversations with many of the elderly regarding the use of exercise to help arthritis etc. This is all fine and dandy on a "normal" basis, however, when I'm in full blown comp mindset, such distractions are just that...a distraction. If you are perfectly fine with training in that situation, then by all means you should consider that facility. If, you are looking to be around more "like minded" people who won't give you a sideways glance as you grunt and throw the weights to the floor, the YMCA might not be for you.

On the other end of the spectrum are the "hard core" gyms. A local gym near my residence is such a place, and one I personally do not feel comfortable working out at even though I AM considered a "hard core" competitor. The gym is basically set up in an oversized garage looking facility, with pieces of equipment that have been around since weight training became popular. The members are made up mainly of guys who wear the string like tank tops and MC Hammer type pants. Many of my male competitor friends love this place. They can grunt, sweat, cuss, throw weights down, and get an "old school" workout. If you are comfortable in that setting, then give it a whirl. I'm sure the place is LOADED with competitors and people who know all about the best exercises to achieve certain results.

Trainers:

Usually your personal trainer will require you attend THEIR place of employment/gym when it comes to personal training. I have seen one or two who will come to your gym for the training, if the gym allows it. Usually you will be required to buy a guest pass for your trainer or be charged a fee of some sort if you bring an outside person in. If you ARE getting frequent PT sessions from the person who is designing your nutrition/workout program, you should highly consider becoming a member of their gym if it fits within all of your requirements.

If you are training at a different facility than the one your PT trains out of, and would still like to use a trainer then having access to one could be of importance. It is very rare (I don't personally know of anyone who does this), but I suppose you could actually hire a PT through the gym to help you get through your workouts designed by your comp prep trainer. Usually trainers have their own method for training, so I'm not sure how well they would take to basically "spotting" you through your workout, but usually money talks so you could always inquire if someone would be willing to do this. I would, however, recommend look into getting a training partner and save your money or simply asking another member to spot you once the weight starts getting too heavy to lift on your own.

Final Note:

If you can find a gym that meets all of your wants and needs then you are good to go. Just remember sometimes, depending on your location and personal circumstances, you might have to prioritize your requirements and choose the one that meets the important ones. If you really need a daycare, and the only gym close by that offers this service doesn't have a wide variety of equipment then you will have to decide which is more important.

Chapter 4

Gym People, the Public, Family and Friends

When you begin your training, it will become obvious to others that you are a girl on a mission. The gym clientele can be broadly categorized to those who are there to casually workout, those that are there to socialize, and those who are there to do some serious training. Being a female, and hitting the weights with intensity and drive, it won't take long for other members to assume you are there with a goal. Once a few weeks pass and your physique has begun to noticeably change, others around you will most certainly know you are serious.

At the beginning, you will most likely offer up the information about your upcoming competition without much prodding. As time goes on, the fatigue sets in, and all you can think about is getting through the workout so you can eat your next meal, you might not be as appreciative of all the inquiring minds. Most of the people are truly intrigued by your changing physique and your dedication; however, there are a few people who could potentially cause a serious issue by talking so much you run out of time to complete your workout. I've noticed most of the people want advice, they want to offer advice, they have questions, or they have concerns. Let's break it down:

People who want advice:

Some guys will approach you asking for "advice" because they want to strike up conversation as more of a pick- up situation. Even if at one point you WERE at the gym in hopes of meeting someone, I can pretty much guarantee your desire to do well at your show is now your number one priority. Handle this situation however you feel comfortable. Just make sure you establish that "now" is not really the time you can discuss.

There will be people who just genuinely want to know what you suggest they do. I've seen it, you've seen it, heck I even was one at one point in my life…the "cardio bunny" as I like to call it. Those are the ladies who really want to look like a competitor but limit their exercise to step aerobics and endless hours on the cardio equipment, not to mention their diets are totally out of sync with what they are trying to accomplish. They see you, they see what you have done and how you've changed in a relatively short amount of time and they want to know how to do it. I don't blame them; I would want to know too! Although I take my training very seriously, I also like helping others when I can.

You can usually give them the basics about the importance of weight training and diet to get them started. However, if they want to know specifics of your plan you should either give them the name and number of your trainer or offer to discuss it with them later. A good way to buy some time is to offer and write out a few "tips" for them when you get home and bring it with you next time you work out. You paid for your program, so how you handle giving that information away for free is a personal decision.

Remember, you are there for a specific reason and can be very polite by simply stating you are on a time schedule and would be more than happy to discuss your training in further over the phone or at a later time. Let me warn you from personal experience, a simple piece of advice can eat up a good hour of your time at the gym thus making for a very long and inter-rupted training session.

They want to offer advice:

Nothing is worse than being in the full midst of your set and someone comes up to you, only to offer advice on how to do the movement different or how another ex-ercise is more effective. It happens, and it will com-pletely interrupt your whole mindset. The biggest group of people who fit into this category is trainers or guys who have weight trained for a significant amount of time.

I do agree that proper form is very important when lift-ing weights, and not suggesting that any advice from a spectator is uncalled for. It only becomes a problem if the person is trying to occupy your time, or using the topic as a means of striking up conversation. If some-one says, "If you curl it a little this way at the top you will feel it better" and then walks on, then consider it genuine advice. If someone wants to spot you, move you to a different exercise, tell you about their training program or anything that keeps you distracted find a polite way to thank them for their concern and tell them you will take it up with your trainer next time you see them.

People who have questions:

People who have questions don't necessarily want advice; they just want to know different things or information. I've been known to stand around talking for a good 20 minutes about the details of my upcoming show, how I'm feeling, what my body fat percentage is, how many abs are showing, and about my vascularity…among other things.

As your competition date gets closer and your body is now reflecting a full blown competitor, people get excited about the impending date. They want to know about your suit, what your diet consists of, how you are feeling and so on. Believe me when I say it is not only possible, but a likelihood you will end up discussing the topic of food for a good amount of time; especially JUNK food. I've been known to have a pretty serious conversation about the different flavors of Oreo's.

Concerned People:

If you have ever stood next to someone who has dieted down, successfully, for a competition you are fully aware of how lean they get. Society, even in the gym, seems to accept a guy sporting single digit body fat;

however become slightly concerned about a female who takes her body down to such levels. Be prepared to be approached by well-meaning gym members who are alarmed at your physical appearance. If they are not familiar with the competition arena and the requirements needed to compete, they will most likely assume you have developed an eating disorder (which will be discussed in the next chapter). Your best approach is to brief them on the ins and outs of competing, assure them you realize it's not necessarily 'healthy,' but that it is also very temporary. Usually you can give them a brief overview of your diet to assure them you ARE eating, and that will suffice. Most people will be amazed you eat 6-7 times a day and able to obtain such a low body fat percentage.

Remember, it is really a compliment that people have become so interested in your progress and training. After all, even though there are a tremendous number of female athletes in this sport, it still seems to be somewhat of an enigma (even in a gym setting) to see a very fit, muscular girl.

The public:

If gym clientele are intrigued by your physique, I'm sure you can imagine what the general public outside of the gym must think. Be prepared to be stopped by complete strangers just about anywhere you go. You might snicker at the idea of this now, but mark my words, you will be asked about your workout regimen, how much you bench, what you eat, and even asked to flex at any given time.

Over the years I've been stopped, while grocery shopping, by complete strangers wanting to know about my diet. One time I was enjoying a cheat meal at a restaurant and a woman came up to my table asking me to flex my arm so she could feel my bicep. As stated above, the elusive, "How much can you bench?" has been asked more than a handful of times. Everyone from mail carriers to waiters to the everyday public will now be interested in what you are doing. At one point, after being stopped by many people, my daughter said, "Do you know ANY of these people?"

Just as there are those who are completely intrigued with your physique, there are others who have a completely different point of view. There are those among the general public who look at a female with a lot of muscle and extremely low body fat as unattractive or unhealthy. I, personally, would never even consider making a rude or catty comment to someone I didn't even know but there are others out there who have no problem with doing so. People who make these comments are usually jealous, feeling self-conscious, or are truly just misinformed about the sport. Consider this as part of your competition journey and take it with a grain of salt.

Family and Friends:

Your family and close friends will likely be the most vocal when it comes to your changing physique. As I stated in Chapter 1, when you tell your family about your plans and how you will be dieting for it, they really have no clue the extent to which you are referring. Most of them will assume you are going to drop a few pounds and maybe (if you mention muscle has anything do with it) throw around a little weight here and there.

After you drop a little body fat, they will comment on how good you are looking. Once you drop a little more, you will start hearing comments like, "You aren't going to lose much more are you?" Once you start closing in on that single digit body fat percentage, they are going to go into a full blown intervention. Be prepared to hear comments like, "You look anorexic," "you are emaciated," and, "this can't be healthy," just to name a few.

You are going to be tired, you are going to be emotional, and the idea of trying to "defend" why you are STILL doing cardio when you are practically "skin and bones" will not be at the top of your to-do list. If you are a first time competitor, I'm certain even YOU are at least a little shocked by the changes you are undergoing and you are aware of the sport's requirements. Your family is most certainly not as informed as you are regarding this, they care for you and your well-being, and should be expected to show some concern.

Once your family/friends start voicing their concerns, you should make it a priority to sit down and address their issues. Explain to them the process and what this sport entails. Reassure them that you understand their concerns; you realize that obtaining such a low body fat might not be the healthiest thing to do, but it is only temporary. Sometimes they just need some perspective and information on the whole subject. Try to reassure them that you are okay and this is just part of your training.

As a preventative measure, once you decide to compete, gather your family/friends around and "warn" them about the journey you are about to undergo and the physical changes you will endure. If you can, find pictures of other competitors, to serve as a great visual and point of reference. Although they will still most likely have concerns once they actually see you go through the changes, this can at least prepare them a little.

Chapter 5
Side Effects

You might be wondering what exactly I mean by "side effects" of competition prep. If this is your first time preparing for a competition, you might be surprised at some of the unexpected side effects of your efforts. If you are going into this believing the only thing you will experience is a lean body, hard muscles, and a phenomenal physique, be prepared…it comes with a price.

Sore Muscles:

Whether or not you are new to lifting weights, you should prepare yourself for many sore days ahead. To build muscles, which is one of your main goals (the other being getting lean), you must first break them down so they can rebuild and become bigger. How do you do that? You lift heavy weights and push your muscles to the point of muscle fatigue. Muscle fatigue is characterized by not being able to complete a full repetition/movement with the weight. By pushing your muscles to this point, you cause micro tears in them, causing them to become damaged and thus repairing them to become larger.

Extreme Tiredness:

You are putting your body through an enormous amount of stress. Not only are you constantly breaking muscles down, but you are also burning a lot of calories through your weight training and cardio. Speaking of calories, depending on where you are at in your training, it is most likely you are running at a calorie deficit each day. Add all of this to your usual daily routine; it's pretty much a guarantee you are going to be dragging through quite a few days.

As I stated at the beginning of the book, sleep is a very important component of your training. In the book, "The Promise of Sleep," written by William C. Dement, M.D.,Ph.D., Dr. Dement notes, "Growth hormone is key, and 'stimulates protein synthesis, helps break down the fats that supply energy for tissue repair, and stimulates cell division to replace old or malfunctioning cells.' If you wish to alter your body's hormonal balance to accelerate recovery and super compensation from your training program, a full night of sleep may again provide the answer."

"As you fall into your deepest phase of sleep-"stage 4" sleep-the quantity of growth hormone released into your bloodstream is increased due to the action of growth hormone-releasing hormone (GHRH). GHRH is itself a sleep inducer, which fits with the suspected function of sleep: a physical state which serves to augment tissue repair, conserve energy, store sugars, and boost the immune system. Conversely, wakefulness appears to reverse these processes, at least in part."

"During waking life, stress hormones are increased, which mobilize sugars for daily activity, in addition to partially suppressing your immune system, and the levels of growth hormone are diminished. Biochemical evidence supports the role of sleep as a critical restorative process, the neglect of which carries a very real physical cost."

You can read the full study at: http://www.bodybuilding.com/fun/hardgainer4.html. So, don't underestimate the importance of sleep; it plays a vital role in your progress!

Insomnia:

No, I haven't lost my mind. I do realize I just stated exhaustion as a side effect, however, insomnia could also prove to be an issue as your training progresses. One cause for this is the impending date of the competition. As the date gets closer, the excitement and nerves of the whole event will keep your mind racing at night which could make for difficulty in falling asleep.

Another cause of sleeplessness is due to overtraining. Wikipedia defines overtraining as the following:

Overtraining is a physical, behavioral, and emotional condition that occurs when the volume and intensity of an individual's exercise exceeds their recovery capacity. They cease making progress, and can even begin to lose strength and fitness. Overtraining is a common problem in weight training, but it can also be experienced by runners and other athletes.

Some of the side effects listed include:

Physiological

Lymphocytopenia

Excessive weight loss

Excessive loss of body fat

Increased resting heart rate

Decreased muscular strength

Increased submaximal heart rate

Inability to complete workouts

Chronic muscle soreness

Fatigue

Increased incidence of injury

Depressed immune system

Constipation or diarrhea

Absence of menstruation

Frequent minor infections/colds

Insomnia

Heart Palpitations

Lower Testosterone Levels

Higher Cortisol Levels

Psychological

Depression

Loss of appetite

Mood Disturbance

Irritability

Loss of motivation

Loss of enthusiasm

Loss of competitive drive

Performance

Early onset of fatigue

Decreased aerobic capacity

Poor physical performance

Inability to complete workouts

Delayed recovery

Night Sweats:

As your training progresses, you could start to experience night sweats. Usually this is caused by fluctuating hormones and/or a boost in your metabolism. As your metabolism becomes more efficient, it fires up within a short time after meal consumption, especially if the meal is high in carbohydrates. If you are consuming your last meal immediately before bed, it is likely you will experience some sweating as a result.

Change in cycle/No period:

There are three basic culprits responsible for infrequent/absent menstrual cycle:

Body fat: In a 1987 study published in "Sports Medicine," researchers debunked the theory that maintenance of body fat percentage of 17 to 22 percent were necessary to maintain normal menstrual function. This same study and others published since then have been unsuccessful in finding a specific cut off point but recognize that low body fat contributes to amenorrhea -- the absence of menstruation.

Exercise: Researchers from Texas A&M and Ball State University estimate the prevalence of infrequent and absent periods to be around 10 and 2 percent, respectively. In athletes, generally those who train for long hours and at high intensities, those numbers increase to 40 and 5 percent, respectively. This suggests that body fat percentage may not be the only factor influencing regular menstrual function.

Diet: Fat cells contribute to nearly 1/3 of estrogen levels in your body. Because of this, low body fat may contribute to low estrogen secretion and subsequent menstrual dysfunction. Low-calorie diets and inadequate nutrition that causes energy deficits are thought to be the primary cause of menstrual dysfunction rather than simple low body fat, according to Dr. Anne Loucks of Ohio University.

Not everyone experiences this symptom during their prep. During one of my prep's I spotted for a month straight, and then lost my cycle completely approximately two months prior to my show. Another time, I lost my period four months prior to my competition. I've also had a season where I didn't lose my period at all, even though I was extremely lean. So, don't be concerned if you DON'T lose it, thinking you might not be lean enough, but on the other hand don't fret if you DO skip a cycle as it is a "normal" side effect.

As a final note on this subject, let me add one final personal experience. I had been training for 13 weeks, was 6 weeks out from my competition, and was very lean. I was not concerned when I missed my period; however I wasn't feeling quite right. Just to be safe I had my husband pick up a pregnancy test. You can imagine my surprise when the word, "Pregnant" appeared. So, if you miss a period and you are feeling "off," it might be a good idea to go ahead and get a test just to rule out a pregnancy.

Extreme Hunger:

When you begin your nutrition plan you might think, "Hey this isn't so bad." Some girls have even commented they can't eat everything they are supposed to eat. Trust me, as time goes on and your metabolism fires into overdrive, the clock will be a main focus. There will be instances where you are ravenous, eat your scheduled meal, and immediately hear the growling of your stomach. This can cause a very uneasy feeling for you mentally, and may even disrupt your sleep in extreme cases. Although the constant hunger is not a pleasant feeling, it can most certainly be expected during your contest prep.

Food obsessions:

This can be especially true for first time competitors who have not yet experienced the nutritional rigor and restriction of competition prep. You must keep in mind that all calories consumed will be the bare minimum of what is required of your body to make the progression that is needed and required in this sport. Taking in 1200 calories a day might not seem overly strict, but when you take into consideration you are burning a good 2000 plus calories a day, the deficit will catch up with you at some point.

As time goes by and you start closing in on the single digit body fat, you might be surprised how often food crosses your mind. About six weeks out from my first competition, I noticed I became obsessed with the Food Network, cookbooks, Bisquick and GrapeNuts. In fact, I once read a cookbook from front to back, making a note of all the recipes I wanted to try once my show was over. I subscribed to numerous cooking magazines, and would make my family elaborate meals just so I could watch them eat. You might think this is over the top (and it could be), but I have many competitor friends who have very similar stories they can tell. The good news is, after your show and a few days of eating anything you can get your hands on, the obsession will start to fade and food commercials won't have the same effect on you as they did prior to your show.

Irritability:

Lack of sleep, constant hunger, extreme fatigue, and ever changing hormones are bound to cause irritability. This alone is enough just cause for your moodiness; however, add a little unseen stressor in your daily routine (like who ate the last of the peanut butter) and you become a ticking time bomb. It is best to accept and admit your edginess and apologize to family and friends ahead of time. I've apologized in advance many days that I woke up feeling "off" and warned my family members of my mood. Don't let your ego or unwillingness to admit your moodiness to those relationships you value cause unneeded extra stress. Try to keep everything in perspective and find a good outlet for your emotions. This too will pass.

Social Isolation:

If you are involved in many social activities or enjoy frequent outings with friends and/or family, there will come a time when going out will seem more of a hassle than worth dealing with. Once the constant hunger and fatigue set in, sitting in a restaurant surrounded by amazing food is not going to be at the top of your "to do" list. Your friends having a swimming party, complete with bar-b-que and drinks? Count yourself out unless standing in the shade (can't get tan lines), drinking water and eating a few ounces of tuna with a half cup of green beans sounds like your idea of a good time.

Unless your friends have competed before, they just cannot comprehend what you are going through. Hearing things like, "Oh this one bite won't hurt you!" and, "Ok, explain to me how having one drink when you are two months out is going to hurt you?" will become frequent conversation. Even well-meaning family members who offer to fix you a meal of egg whites will have to be reminded that ham, sausage, cheese, and other ingredients do not constitute an acceptable form of competition fare.

Lastly, if all the above were not reason enough to avoid public events, the sheer effort it will take to attend will seem too much. During prep, your meals will need to be eaten at scheduled time. If you will be attending a wedding and reception for a few hours, you best plan on packing a cooler filled with enough meals to get you through the event. Eating meals on schedule (remember the extreme hunger topic?) will be your highest priority; anything that threatens your meal timing will not be given second thought.

Frequent Urination:

Get ready to know the exact location of every bathroom within your traveling vicinity. It is usual practice for trainers to require a minimum of a gallon of water to be drank each day. You will become accustomed to scheduling bathroom usage into your daily routine. Things like a simple grocery store trip will include using the bathroom before you leave and locating it within the grocery store upon arrival. I should also add that your days of drinking from a glass will come to an end, being replaced by a gallon jug. As a tip, try getting most/all of your water consumed a couple hours prior to bed time or else plan on waking up a few times for middle of the night bathroom trips.

Constipation:

This most likely will not become an issue until later in competition prep. As your body becomes more efficient in burning every single calorie and consuming every little nutrient, there won't be a lot of extra "waste" for your body to dispose of. Usually the problem can be solved by incorporating some healthy fats (or fat supplements) into your diet, or if all else fails a natural fiber based laxative like Metamucil will do the trick. It's always important to discuss this with your trainer to assess the situation and determine the best action to take.

Final Notes:

These are some of the main "side effects" of your training and nutrition program, although other perfectly normal ones might also pop up such as muscle cramps and loss of feeling/tingling in extremities (due to pinched nerves). On the other hand, there is nothing "wrong" if you don't experience any/all of the symptoms listed above. As with anything, if you are experiencing something that you are not quite sure if it is "normal" or not, seek the advice of your trainer or a medical professional.

Chapter 6

It's all in the details!

Your training is well under way, your body is starting to change, and the competition date is approaching. As I'm sure you are aware, the competition preparation encompasses other aspects above and beyond simply training and dieting. No matter what category you are competing in, there are certain details that need to be taken care of before stepping on stage. Do not be quick to dismiss these as "small" details, as they can have a significant impact on your placement come show time.

Do your homework:

If you have never been to a competition, then you should strongly consider trying to attend a local show to observe how it is run and to take note of what is expected. Actually witnessing a competition can be a wealth of information. You will get a good idea of how girls are lined up, what physiques are winning, what suit color/cuts look best on stage, different poses, and so on.

Online sites dedicated to competition coverage and bodybuilding can also be a good resource. There are numerous sites and forums designated primarily for discussions regarding competition prep and offer a tremendous amount of information on anything and everything to do with the subject. A wealth of information can be found at bodybuilding.com, including personal blogs and journals of competitors who make their journey open to the public. Typing key words like, "competition prep," "mandatory poses for women's physique," "figure poses" and so on will also provide an array of helpful sites.

Posing:

As far as contest prep goes, this can be considered your number one make or break point outside of your conditioning. In fact, I've witness numerous girls who have amazing physique, but have not given ample practice time to their posing and thus could not properly display their hard work on stage. As one of my close friends, who happens to be a judge, stated, "You can have a great physique, but if you don't know how to show it, we can't see it and we don't have time to wait while you try to figure it out." Consider learning and perfecting your poses of upmost priority, allowing plenty of time to practice.

Posing Coach:

Although it is possible to learn the different poses by watching a show or looking at pictures, you would be well served to consider hiring a posing coach. A posing coach can be anyone who is very familiar with the sport, knowledgeable of the required poses YOU will need to perform, and understands what the judges are looking for…right down to the smallest of details.

As with many things, the most reliable and direct source would be to ask another competitor who helps them with their posing. Just as trainers/nutritionists become well known in the bodybuilding community, a good posing coach can also be found. Usually your trainer will have some feedback regarding a person to contact, or offer their services as an option. Usually the coach is a local competitor who has been very successful in competitions or even a judge who offers posing classes in their spare time.

Remember, it is very important to enlist the help of someone who is familiar with the poses you will be required to show. If the posing coach is a figure competitor and has never done bikini, they might not be the most qualified in helping you with your bikini poses. However, if they are figure competitor and have trained other bikini girls, successfully, with their poses then they will work just fine.

Most coaches have an hourly rate, and will leave the frequency of the meetings up to you. Some also offer a group rate, which is usually cheaper than a private session, where you run through poses in a group. Both methods are effective and can be decided based on your personal preference.

The posing can be divided into two (sometimes three) sections: symmetry, mandatories (Fitness, Bodybuilding and Women's Physique), and freestyle.

Symmetry:

Although symmetry is important in every category, it is singled out and prevalent in Figure, Fitness, Women's Physique, and Bodybuilding. Depending on the judges, symmetry is often considered the number one criteria in determining placements and always within the top three considerations (along with conditioning and muscle tone).

Symmetry by definition is the correspondence in size, form, and arrangement of parts on opposite sides of a plane. In relation to bodybuilding, this simply means that your right side should be as developed as your left, your front should be as developed as your back and your upper body should be as developed as your lower body.

All categories display symmetry by performing quarter turns. You will be asked to face the judges, and then asked to "quarter turn" in which case you will turn to the right, displaying your side. During the next quarter turn you will now have your backside facing the judges. The third turn will display your right side; the final turn will have you back to your starting point facing the judges.

Although the symmetry round is based on the same quarter turns for all categories, be aware of the rules that differ from organization to organization on how you present them. The front and back pose is universal, however, the side poses differ slightly depending on which federation you are competing in. The NPC does not allow any twisting of the body when you display your side; your hands and arms must stay down to your side with your torso staying square to the rest of your body. The NANBF allows the competitor to twist their torso, keeping hips facing forward but shoulders and chest turned slightly towards the judges with the arm closest to judges extending backwards and arm furthest away coming forward. Make sure your posing coach is aware of the different style allowed.

Mandatories:

If you are competing in Figure, you do not have mandatory poses outside of the symmetry round of quarter turns. However, if you are competing in Fitness, Physique or Bodybuilding, you will also be judged based on mandatory poses. Again, make sure your coach is well versed in how to properly display these poses and knows exactly which poses will be asked of you. It is not enough to say, "Ok, double bicep is like this." If you are working with someone knowledgeable enough, they will be able to give you tips such as, "Twist your hand this way to make the peak come out," and, "make sure you are flexing your leg this way while doing that pose."

Fitness competitors present their mandatory poses during their fitness routine. The mandatory moves include: one arm push up, straddle hold, leg extension hold, full split front, high kick, and full split-side. These can be done in any order during the routine, as long as all of them are included.

Even though Women's Physique and Bodybuilding are similar in their mandatories, there is a huge difference in how they are performed. A physique competitor will display a front double bicep by keeping hands open, where as a bodybuilder will display the same pose by making a fist. Don't dismiss these subtle differences as insignificant; they are major judging criteria between the categories.

The Physique mandatories consist of: front double bicep, side chest, side tricep, back double bicep, and abdominals. Unlike bodybuilding, all poses are to be performed very fluid, feminine, and with open hands at all times. There is also no "set" way to display these poses. Some girls display their front double biceps by extending a leg and pointing their toes while facing judges, others turn to the side and twist their upper body towards the judges. A qualified posing coach will know this and help you display your body/poses in a way that flatters you the most.

Bodybuilding mandatories consist of: front double bicep, front lat spread, side chest, side tricep, rear double bicep, rear lat spread, and abdominals/thigh. Sometimes the judges will also ask for most muscular and/or favorite pose. Unlike Physique, there is no requirement to keep hands open and most are done with a closed fist. There is also usually a uniform way to display each pose.

Freestyle:

This is prevalent in the Figure division and is also sometimes called the "model walk/T walk." This is usually performed after the symmetry round in the NANBF and before symmetry in the NPC. You will be asked to come onto the stage, by yourself, and will walk to one side of the stage where you will perform a couple poses of your choice. You will then walk to the other side of the stage and hit another couple poses. Usually the process is concluded by walking center stage, hitting a final pose or two, waving "good bye" to the audience and exiting the stage. Usually these poses are chosen based on what makes your physique looks the best and are solely up to the competitor. If your butt or backside is not a strong point, there is no rule stating you MUST show your back during the freestyle portion. Bikini competitors have somewhat of a mesh of symmetry, mandatories, and freestyle all thrown together. For instance, when showing their backside to show symmetry (and which is also somewhat of a mandatory), they have personal freedom to hit that pose with as much flair and personal preference as they want. Also, unlike other competitors, it is perfectly acceptable for bikini competitors to look back over their shoulder at the judges when displaying their back.

Again, having a posing coach who is well versed in what will be expected of you can save a lot of time and worry. Being familiar with each pose as well as being able to properly display those poses can make a HUGE difference in how well you fare in the line-up. If you are slow to hit your poses, or standing next to someone who is nailing their poses, you are only going to make them look better and make yourself look worse. Remember, you have a very short amount of time in front of the judges, and most have a good idea of the physique you are bringing, within the first minute on stage. Learn your poses and then practice them until you could do them in your sleep.

Choreographer:

If you are competing in Fitness, Physique or Bodybuilding you will be required to perform a routine. The routine will be done to a song of your choice and is usually approximately 60-90 seconds long; this varies from show to show and can be found in the rules section of your entry form. During your routine you will have total freedom to hit any and all poses you would like. There are no set rules on what has to be done, but is usually a combination of mandatory poses and dance like transitions.

Fitness is also done to music, but is mainly focused on performing gymnastic movements such as pushups, flips, and jumps; whereas Physique and Bodybuilding routines are filled with mandatory poses.

A choreographer can be a great resource, if like me; you really have no idea how to come up with your own routine. Once you find someone who is willing to put a routine together for you, they will probably request a copy of the song that will be used. After the routine is complete, a time will be scheduled to run through it. It is always a good idea to video the choreographer as they perform it, so you can watch it at home or whenever you are trying to learn the moves. Like a posing coach, choreographers usually charge by the hour and leave the number of sessions up to the competitor based on their needs.

I know plenty of girls who choreographed their own routines and had great success. If you are confident of your ability to put a routine together, then by all means go for it! There is no rule about hiring outside help, and the judges have no clue if you enlisted help or did it on your own. As long as the routine is fluid and consistent and you are confident with the end result, that is all that matters.

Stage Presence:

All categories, especially Bikini, Figure, Fitness and Women's Physique are also judged on stage presence. This is broad category and encompasses many smaller details which add to the overall picture. Some of the qualities include: hair, make up, overall appearance, jewelry, skin tone, personality, confidence, and flow (how you move as you hit poses and walk in heels.) Basically anything that has to do with how you display your overall package is considered in stage presence.

Chapter 7
Suit(s)

You've chosen your show, your training is well under way, and you are practicing your posing on a daily basis. It's now time to start your search for a suit to wear on the big day. If you have never done any research on a competition suit, you might not realize all the details which need to be considered when picking one out.

I have been selling suits for approximately seven years, and in that time have noticed a trend of questions among competitors; especially first time ones. When talking to a client, the first thing I ask is, "Are you familiar with the average cost of a suit?" I've come to realize that although girls know they can be pricey, they might not be aware of just how expensive they can be. The suit is also among the top three expenses you will incur and if you aren't prepared for this, you could experience a little bit of "sticker shock" when the time comes to purchase one. With price being the number one concern among girls purchasing a suit, they also have follow-up questions/concerns. Let's address them individually.

Cost:

Usually competitors aren't quite sure why a suit costs as much as it does. After all, there really isn't much material required for one yet the price can range from $300-$2000, so why the huge discrepancy? Many factors are considered when determining the final selling price. Some of the main factors are: designer, type of stones being used, how many stones being used, and the time required to design the suit.

Designer:

When I began competing, I purchased my first suit from someone who is now a very well-known designer, but was just starting out back then. The suit I purchased was moderately stoned and cost $300. Although time and inflation to play into price increases, this designer became very sought after among the pros and her prices changed to reflect the demand. I recently looked on her site, finding a very similar suit as the one I had purchased, being listed for around $600. Bottom line is if you are using a designer who has been in the business for quite a while and is accustomed to suiting up the top names in the industry, be prepared to pay a decent amount for their service.

On the other hand, do not be quick to dismiss small or private designers. I, admittedly, do not publicly advertise my services and sell only via online sites, referral, or repeat customers. This does not mean I'm not qualified to provide a high quality suit, but merely reflects the fact that I do not care to become so busy I cannot do anything outside stoning suits all day. I also limit my business in order to provide more personal service and allow plenty of attention to each individual suit, without feeling overwhelmed.

Over the years I have seen many individuals, most are competitors, get into the business of providing suits. I've seen pictures of their suits and must say they can be just as elaborate and beautiful as any of the "established" businesses. A bonus to a smaller business or personal designer is that the cost of a suit is usually lower, due to less overhead.

Do not get me wrong, there are many larger, well established businesses out there that have been in business for a long time due to the fact they offer high quality suits and reasonable prices. The great thing about a well-known business is that they have earned their reputation, their suits are consistent, and they usually have more of a variety of designs and materials to choose from. My point is merely not to dismiss a suit or a designer based on the fact they don't make suits for a living. Consider all options and make informed choices based on the criteria you are looking for.

Rhinestones vs. Crystals:

One of the main things I've seen affect the price of a suit is the type of stones being used. As an example: A girl had been sent to me by her trainer to purchase a suit. She found one online she liked and asked me for a quote. When I quoted a price that was about $150 more than the online price, she thanked me for my time and said she would just get it from the site. I told her I understood, but cautioned her to read the description of the suit and the stones being used due to the pricing of the suit. She wrote back and said, "They use rhinestones." I explained to her the difference between a rhinestone and the stones I used; in the end she purchased the suit from me and followed up with a letter stating she received numerous compliments on the suit at her show.

Rhinestones are defined as a small fake gem: a small piece of paste or glass used as an imitation diamond. The definition alone should clue you into the quality it provides. Imagine being on stage and your suit is stoned with "a small piece of paste or glass." I'm sure you an easily picture how much (or little) shine the stone is going to emit… not a lot.

I've also had girls seek me out, in a panic, due to a suit they received being designed with rhinestones that actually looked more plastic than anything. If you are considering an amazing priced suit that is adorned with a significant amount of stones, be sure to check what type of stone is being used (this is also a good question to ask designers). The saying, "You get what you pay for" is prevalent in this situation.

Crystals:

When searching for your suit, be sure to ask/verify the stones being used are crystals. Although there are many different brands of crystals, the absolute best one available is the Swarovski Crystal.

Swarovski is the brand name for a range of cut crystal and related luxury products produced by Swarovski AG of Wattens, Austria. They are specifically cut/designed to allow the best shine and brilliance under the stage lights. The amount of shine and sparkle they emit once the lights hit them cannot be rivaled.

Just as a suit designer that is well established charges more for their services, having your suit stoned with a product from the number one provider of crystals used in "luxury products" will also drive the cost up. If you are interested in using different shapes and/or colors of crystals on your suit, you should expect to pay even more. Although the crystals are a little more expensive than rhinestones, it is not a night and day difference in cost compared to the difference you will see on stage. The choice always comes down to your personal cost budget; however, I would suggest sacrificing a few rhinestones to allow for a smaller amount of crystals to be used. Just be knowledgeable in what you purchase so that you won't be disappointed once you receive your suit.

Number of stones being used:

This topic is pretty much self-explanatory and doesn't need much discussion. If you are looking at a suit design that uses 200 stones, it is obviously not going to cost as much as one containing 2000 stones. Again, you must also factor in any colored or different shaped crystals into the overall price of the suit.

Time required for design:

Some designs are very intricate and require a decent amount of time and skill when being put on a suit. Other designs are more basic, use less stones, and can be done fairly quickly. It is pretty apparent by looking at a suit, the amount of time and skill needed to complete the design. As with the number of crystals being used, the amount of time required for your suit to be completed will be a factor in the pricing.

Budgets and Negotiation:

If you are purchasing a pre-designed suit from a

business, chances are the price is set. Usually a picture of the suit, an explanation of the stones used, and the selling price will be shown on the site and you will be able to purchase the suit via an online shopping cart method. I refer to these types of suits as "mass produced" suits and available to as many people that wish to purchase them.

However, if you are purchasing a custom suit from a designer, meaning they are making it specifically for you and not based on a "mass produced" design, you will have more flexibility in the pricing. All the above factors such as number of stones, time required, and intricacy of the design will be taken into account. Sometimes you can negotiate a price with the designer in custom design situations. If they offer to design it for $400, it would not be out of the question for you to ask if they could consider doing the suit for $350. Don't expect to negotiate a price too far off from the price they have quoted.

Another way to purchase a custom suit is based on a pre-set budget. When I'm dealing with girls interested in ordering a suit, I give them the option of setting a budget for me to work within and allow limited input into the design. If a girl has set aside $400 for a suit, I will either show her a few stone designs that fall into her budget, or get an overall idea of what she likes (swirls, straight lines, etc.) and stone the suit based on her budget. I've also had girls email me pictures of suits they like and ask me to make a similar design that fit into their allotted budget. Usually you will have more options regarding budget and negotiations when you work with a private seller or in purchasing a custom suit.

Payments:

Most people don't have an extra $500 just lying around and become concerned about how to pay for a suit. Paying for the suit over a set amount of payments is sometimes offered, depending on the designer and their policies. Sometimes a non-refundable deposit is required to begin designing the suit (usually half of total cost), with the remaining amount due to be paid in full before the suit is handed over. Some designers require payment in full upon ordering. If you want to be able to make payments, be sure to check with the designer on their policy regarding payments.

Refunds and Returns:

I don't speak on behalf of every suit designer, but usually refunds are out of the question. We understand that things happen, emergencies arise, and sometimes girls decide they just don't want to compete anymore.

Although we are sympathetic to those issues, it really isn't OUR fault your circumstances have changed. We have purchased the material, paid for the crystals, spent hours designing it, and have handed the suit over. Just because you are no longer in need of the suit has no bearing on the fact we have spent numerous resources on producing it for you. Your best bet is to try to sell the suit to another competitor. Returns are usually more flexible, but limited. I, personally, allow exchanges on custom suits, but only for a replacement of the correct size of the exact same suit design. Some designer's state very specifically they do not allow exchanges on suits, period, while others will exchange for the exact suit on the correct size if returned within a certain number of days of purchase. If the suit shows obvious signs of wear or is exchanged after a significant amount of time, chances are you will be stuck with your original purchase. As always, ask the designer if they offer refunds or what their policy is regarding exchanges.

Material:

Choosing the color of material you wish to have your suit made from is an important and personal decision. If you are completely unsure of what color to go with, most designers are willing to give you an opinion on what would look best. A good rule of thumb is to look at the color of clothing you wear, and observe which colors look best on you. Some designers offer to send fabric samples (usually for a price) that you can put up against your skin to get a better visual. As with other things, using the internet to look at competitors with similar coloring (hair, eyes, skin tone) and observing the color of suit they are wearing, can be extremely helpful.

Not only are suits available in multiple colors, they also come in different types of material, including Lycra, velvet, foil, and hologram. The type of material you want wear is another personal choice, but seems to follow a trend. When I started competing, velvet was the main material used for a suit. Fast forward seven years later, foils and holograms are now prevalent with velvet being almost extinct. As in life, clothing is personal to the person wearing it; just because it is a trend doesn't mean you HAVE to follow. Pick what you feel most confident in, and looks the best on your body.

You've picked out the color and the material; next up is the size and cut of suit. The size and cut of suit are the two most important factors when ordering. Whereas the color and type of material are a completely personal choice, the correct cut/size is an absolute requirement above all else. You can have a beautifully designed suit, but if the suit doesn't fit you right it won't matter if there is 1 or 1000 stones on it, you are going to be disappointed and most likely judged, during show time, accordingly. I've seen many girls who have amazing physiques, but wore a suit that was too big or cut wrong for their body type, and thus totally threw off their whole appearance on stage.

The number one tendency among females, especially those who have a little more "junk in the trunk" so to speak is to cover their backside with a larger or wider cut suit bottom. Let me warn you against this. If you cover your rear end with a wider cut/larger suit, all the judges are going to see when they look at you is a whole lot of material. Not only is this distracting, but it actually makes your backside look worse than a narrower cut bottom. Believe me; you are not fooling anyone by trying to "cover" your rear end.

As far as the top is concerned, the tendency here is to also go bigger than necessary. If you have too much material on your chest, chances are your lats will be covered and your chest will not look as wide or open as it should. The top of your suit should cover your breasts only, not your lats and collar bone. If you are planning on wearing inserts in your top, make sure you inform the designer of this as the top will need to be made a tad larger than your "natural" size in order to allow room for the insert.

On the opposite end of being too large, is of course picking a suit in a size that is too small. Most organizations specifically state on their site and entry form that thongs are not allowed. You will be asked to bring your suit to registration for inspection to ensure it meets the width requirements. If you try to wear a thong on stage, chances are you will not be allowed to compete. As far as the top is concerned, there is nothing wrong with a little bit of the inside of your breast to be visible, however, if you are close to falling out or exposing areola, you can expect to be judged down. Just remember families and children usually attend these shows, so keep it as classy as possible without draping yourself in excess material.

How far out should I look for suit?

You can begin looking for a suit as soon as you decide to compete; however you probably don't need to purchase until approximately 6-8 weeks out from your show. Although you do not need to be "stage ready" when you order your suit, you will need to have a good idea of what your estimated competition weight will be.

Most suits are made from a 4-way stretch material and allow for a good 10 pound variance. When you order your suit, the designer will most likely need your height, cup size, and estimated competition weight. If you are working with a trainer, they will be your number one resource in determining what weight they expect you to compete at. As long as they have a good idea of this weight, within a 10 pound range, you should have no problem ordering the correct suit size. Another consideration will be how your weight is distributed. I've worn the same size bottom weighing 110, as I did when I weighed 120, but the weight gain was due to muscle distribution over my whole body thus did not affect my waist size. In order to allow for this discrepancy, some designers will require you to measure certain points on your body or send a picture of yourself so they can better gauge your body composition. All designers understand you are not at your show weight when ordering and have allowed for this when helping you determine the correct size; allowing you to order well in advance of your competition.

Do I need more than one suit?

The answer to this is, "it depends." If you are a bodybuilder, you will most likely want two suits. The prejudging section does not allow multi-colored or stoned suits. This means you will not be allowed to wear any hologram material or have a stone design of any sort. However, at the night show you are allowed to wear any color suit with as many stones as you wish. Some ladies prefer to have a prejudging suit as well as a more elaborate night show suit; whereas some are fine with wearing the morning show suit in the evening portion. There is no set rule about having to wear a different suit in the finals and can be left up to your personal choice.

If you are in Bikini, Figure, or Women's Physique you are allowed to wear the same suit for prejudging and the evening show. There is nothing wrong with taking a suit as a "back up" if you feel the need, but there is no rule for or against it. It is common practice for girls to wear their morning show suit for the night show and less common to change the suit out in between.

If you are in Fitness, you will be required to wear a fitness suit for your routine. Most of the suits consist of boy cut shorts and a top that exposes the arms, midriff, and back, and represent some sort of theme. I've seen "costumes" that represent Superwoman, a "biker chick," and a referee. Usually the outfit is based on the song being used for the routine, although this is not a must.

Can I wear the same suit to multiple shows?

Absolutely! There is no need to purchase a new suit for every single show. Although the suit is critical for your competition, you must remember it is the fit and cut of the suit that is of upmost importance. If you have purchased a suit that looks amazing on your physique, then by all means stick with it until you decide you just want to purchase a different one. Judges see hundreds, if not thousands, of girls every week. They do not remember every single suit worn and who actually wore it. Even if by some slight chance the judges do remember you wearing that suit, you are not docked in any sort of way unless the suit was not a good fit/cut the first time around.

Buy vs. Rent:

When I began competing, there wasn't really anywhere to rent a suit. Over the years, a few companies and private sellers have offered rental suits as a solid option. This can be a great way to get a suit for a fraction of the cost and is ideal for girls who aren't sure they are going to compete in the future or are on a strict budget.

Rental prices can be a set price or can vary depending on the level of intricacy of the suit. Almost all rental suits are used suits and have been worn multiple times, and come only in the size listed. Each designer offering rental suits has different policies regarding price and how long you will be allowed to keep the suit. Be sure to read their policy regarding cost, when you can get the suit, how long you can keep the suit, and damage protection.

As a final note, most rental prices are about 1/3 to ½ of the total purchase price of the suit. If you are certain you will be competing in more than one show, it might be more cost effective to actually purchase a suit and sell it when you are ready to purchase another one or are done competing.

New vs. Used:

Of course the obvious benefit of purchasing a new suit is that it has never been worn. You don't have to worry about stains, tears, missing stones, or obvious wear and tear on the suit. There is something to say for feeling confident about the product you are going to receive, knowing you won't be in for any "surprises" regarding its condition. The biggest "downside" is cost; you can expect to pay more for a suit that has never been worn.

Do not dismiss the option of purchasing a used suit, as they are usually sold by competitors at a fraction of what they originally purchased it for. Just because a suit is used, does not mean you can expect a damaged or less than perfect suit. Many girls take very good care of their suit and ensure it stays in great condition.

The absolute best place (as of right now) to purchase a used suit is online at www.divaexchange.com . The site is dedicated to selling two piece suits, bikini's, fitness wear, evening gowns, shoes, and even jewelry. At any given time you can look on the site and have a plethora of suits to choose from.

The suits are listed by categories (Figure, Bikini, Fitness, etc) and include pictures of the suit being sold. There is a brief description of the suit, including the size, condition, stones used, price, and the sellers contact information. Almost all sellers are willing to negotiate their selling price, even on suits that are listed at half of their original cost.

Be certain to verify the condition of the suit, including missing stones, tears and stains. The prices are usually so reasonable, the sellers are more than open about any flaws the suit might have. It's just always best to verify all information regarding the suit, including the stats, as most do not offer returns once they mail it out to you.

Also consider Diva Exchange as a resource if you are looking for a new suit. Many small or private designers (including me) use the site as a method of selling ALL suits, including brand new ones. The best part is that new listings are being put up every single day, so make sure you check back on a frequent basis.

When you are ready to part with your suit, you can easily list it on Diva and get exposure from all over the world. As of right now, the cost to list a suit on the site is approximately $4 for a 30 day listing, but can vary based on number of photos included and length of time you want to list. Consider this site your number one shopping portal if you are on a tight budget.

Resources:

Here are a list of resources regarding purchasing or renting a suit. Each company offers different services and not all offer rentals. Some also do not offer suits for all categories, so be sure to check each one out and chose based on what best fits your needs. *I do not claim any one designer to be better or more highly qualified than another, and claim NO RESPONSIBILITY regarding any product you might receive by using their service. This is simply a resource for you providing different (not all) options available to you in your search for a suit.*

www.Cherrybombs.net

www.DivaExchange.com

www.suitsyouswimwear.com

www.passionfruitdesigns.com

www.jagware-posingsuits.com

www.tameemarie.webs.com

Chapter 8
Miscellaneous Purchases

Now that you have purchased your suit, or are at least knowledgeable about purchasing one, you can turn your attention to rounding up some miscellaneous items. As I stated at the beginning of the book, this sport definitely comes with a cost, and not a cheap one at that. Sometimes all the little "odd and ends" can really start to add up. If you wait until last minute to start purchasing everything, it might put more of a financial strain on you than if you slowly start getting things you need.

Shoes:

The only categories that do not require heels are Women's Physique and Bodybuilding. If you are competing in anything besides those two, you are going to need to purchase some heels. Most girls opt for a clear shoe, approximately 4"-5" tall. Shoes are a personal preference regarding which style you choose to go with. Some options available are: ankle straps, platforms, crystals, height, and color. Shoes can be purchased via many of the suit sites listed in the previous chapter as well as www.snaz75.com .

When choosing your shoes, make sure you pick a style

and height you will feel most comfortable walking and posing in. Part of your stage presence is judged on how well you move in those shoes. I've actually witnessed a competition where the judges were having such a hard time deciding between two girls for the overall, that they simply asked the competitors to walk back and forth on the stage. One girl walked very confidently in her shoes, while the other one sort of "clomped" across the stage. Needless to say, the girl who looked most comfortable in her heels displayed the better stage presence and thus won the show. During your time on stage, you will be required to walk, stop, hit poses and move in a way that appears effortless. Also keep in mind that bodybuilders have most likely been on stage prior to you and have left traces of oil right where you will be walking. If you have ever witnessed a girl slip on stage, you understand that she stands out like a sore thumb, enticing a collective gasp among the audience. If you are a tennis shoe or flip flop girl like I am, be sure to allow ample time to become comfortable in your heels. As I was told during my first show, "You need to look like you are capable of mowing the lawn in those heels." So, be sure to practice and then practice some more; you will be glad you did.

Jewelry:

If you are in bodybuilding, you are not allowed to wear jewelry to prejudging. All other categories are not only allowed to wear jewelry to the morning show, but highly encouraged to do so. Keep in mind that you are being judged based on your overall appearance, and jewelry plays a significant part in that illusion.

The main pieces of jewelry to consider are: earrings, rings, and bracelets. I purposefully left the necklace out of the list. Part of your body you are being judged on is your chest; if you have a necklace covering your chest it will be difficult to see that body part. I've seen girls opt for a choker and still place well; however, I found it to be highly distracting and noticed it seemed to disrupt the whole flow of their upper body.

As far as your other jewelry is concerned, there is no set standard on what is acceptable, although the usual trend includes attributes such as being big and shiny. If you want jewelry that matches your suit, then go for it. Just make sure you sparkle under the lights and choose items that are not too over the top or distracting. If you are considering a tiara just make sure you have the personality to pull it off. Another option to consider would be shiny bobby pins, barrettes, clips, and/or hair bands. Remember: classy not distracting.

Hair:

If you're not sporting your natural hair color, you will need to make sure and schedule a haircut/trim and color touch up before show time. The best time to plan on getting your hair tended to would be the week of the show, allowing plenty of time to work with it. If you get your color touched up too far out from the competition, you risk having visible roots come time for the big day. Within the hair topic, is the discussion of hair extensions, curly or straight, and the ever popular, "should I wear it up or down?" question. If you are considering wearing hair extensions, be sure you choose wisely. There are so many different options available including clip- in, ponytail extenders, and professional extensions. Whichever route you go, be sure your hair looks natural and "classy," and by all accounts, give yourself plenty of time to work with your extensions so you will feel confident in whatever style you end up going with.

In regards to the question, "curly or straight," this is also a personal decision. There is no absolute right way to go when it comes to your hair. The overall goal regarding EVERYTHING about your look is to make sure it is what looks best on YOU and portrays the look you are shooting for. If your hair looks good with a few curls in it, then by all means put them in there. If you look best with straight hair, then go that route. I've personally worn my hair in both fashions, usually making the final decision the morning of the show. The hair up vs. down is open for debate. I was told by a judge, that you should either have really short hair as in a pixie cut or other sassy style, or have long hair. The in-between length of hair is the "gray" area, and you should consider the use of extensions. Again there is no rule on this, but I did ask her personal opinion as a judge, what was preferred. I was also told that wearing your hair down also seemed to have a pull among the judges, but if you wanted to pull a few strands back away from your face, or leave some up and some down, that was also an option. Let me clarify that you will not be judged down because you pulled your hair into a pony tail, just remember it's about being feminine and looking well put together. If all else fails, try putting your hair in different styles and have your trainer or a friend/family give you feedback on what flatters you most.

Nails:

To me, wearing fake nails is the worst part of the whole prep because I have a really hard time functioning with them on. In fact, I postpone getting my nails until just a couple days out from the show. Whether or not you are used to wearing nails, you will need to consider getting them prior to your show. The only girls who can get away with not wearing them are the bodybuilders, but even then I'm pretty certain they still get a good manicure beforehand.

I admit, I despise nails so much that I've actually worn the press on nails during a competition. Although they worked just fine, I had to make sure and take extra nails and glue with me just in case they popped off. If you decide to just stick some on, be sure to apply them right before you leave for your show to ensure they stay on, and always take back up nails and glue!

Do not forget your toes! There are some great press on toe nails available, which I have used for all but one of my shows over the past seven years. They look natural, stay on well, and are fairly cheap. If you do not want to fuss with the press on nails, you should consider getting a pedicure when you are getting your fingernails done. If you are talented enough, there are some great do-it-yourself French manicure sets available for you to apply yourself. It really doesn't matter what you do to make your toes look pretty, just remember that your shoes are open toed, and your feet will be seen.

Makeup:

If you look back through the judging criteria at the beginning of the book, you will see that "attractiveness" is listed as one element you are judged on. I'm sure you can guess that the main source of your appearance, besides your physique, is your face…or more specifically…your make up. I'm sure you have seen pictures of beautifully tanned competitors who's face appears about three shades lighter, thus giving an illusion of a cut and paste head on a body.

When you get tanned (or apply your own tan), you will either have only one light coat of tanning solution on your face or none at all, therefore you will need to make sure you allow for this discrepancy by purchasing a foundation that matches your overall tan. The brand of foundation is not of huge importance; however you need to consider its "staying power" under the bright lights. MAC cosmetics do offer a stage make up that is amazing at handling the heat and bright lights, although it is a little more expensive than something like Cover Girl.

When purchasing your makeup, keep in mind that you will be standing under bright, hot, unforgiving lights. All makeup needs to be applied darker than what you would ever be caught dead wearing in public, yet appear glamorous on stage. If you are concerned about applying your makeup, you can always enlist the help of a friend/competitor or hire a makeup artist to help you. Most shows do offer hair and makeup services, for a price, to those competitors who might not want to mess with doing it themselves. Usually the "official" makeup artist is listed on the show website, Facebook page, or on the entry form. If you are unsure if one is available or not, you can contact the show promoters. Be sure to book well in advance, as I know many girls use this service and space is limited.

Photo Shoot:

There is almost always an official photographer associated with the show. Their information is also usually found the same place as the makeup artist. You need to keep in mind that although booking a photo shoot is not a necessity, you are going to look your absolute best during this time and will most likely want some sort of photographic memento. Most photographers are very diligent about promoting their services and will inform you how to order pictures from the show or how to book a private shoot. Private shoots, especially with well-known photographers, book up very quickly so don't put this off until the last minute. For more information regarding photo shoots, please see the Q and A section (located at the end of the book) with professional photographer, Doug Jantz.

Tanning:

All shows usually have a designated tanning company they have enlisted for the competition. A good "estimated" cost to enlist their service is approximately $100, and worth every single penny. Not only do they ensure your tan looks even and flawless, but they do touch ups at any given time throughout the show. Coming from someone who used to do the whole tanning thing in my home, this saves a TON of time, worry, and mess! If you can afford this expense, you will not be disappointed. Be sure to book well ahead of time, as most competitors now use these services in lieu of applying the tan themselves.

Each company usually provides you with a list of things you need to do prior to getting tanned. It is not uncommon for them to require exfoliation of the skin the whole week prior to the show. Also, if you were not aware, you will need to shave your body from neck to feet approximately 1-2 days prior to tan application. Again, you can expect to get a list of these procedures as well as others upon booking your tan time.

As a side note to tanning, I often get asked if it is

necessary to get a base tan, from a tanning bed, prior to show time. I've got mixed feelings on this, but will tell you what the "norm" is. Most competitors DO spend some time in the tanning bed to establish some sort of base tan. It is believed that due to the intensity of the stage lights, you can appear somewhat washed out if you do not have a good base tan. I, personally, have always hit the tanning bed approximately 6-8 weeks out from my show. With that being said, I also have friends who absolutely refuse to step foot in a tanning bed, have opted to only get the spray tan, and didn't experience any issues at all.

Food cooler:

Although I'm certain you feel as if you don't get to eat at all and are on the brink of starvation, rest assured you will be packing plenty of food to take to your show. Competitions last a very long time, and it will be imperative that you have plenty of food to get you through pre-judging. Invest in a medium size food cooler that is easy to tote around, yet will hold a decent amount of food. Although possible to pack your food in the same bag containing all your other competition things, it just makes for less hassle and mess to have your food in a separate location that is easily accessible.

Competition bag:

If you do not own a piece of luggage, preferably with wheels, comparable to a carry on you will need to purchase one. Everything you used in your personal preparation (brush, makeup, curling iron, hairspray, shoes etc) will be taken with you to the show to allow for touch-up if needed. Again, depending on what category you are in, you could have two hours or more before you ever step on stage. The best way to allow for this, and to ensure you look stage ready when your time comes, is to have access to anything you might need for a touch up. If your curls go flat before you are called to be judged, the curling iron will do you no good if it is setting at home in the bathroom. When in doubt...pack it! (Details about what to pack will be discussed later).

Chapter 9
Entry Form

Once you have decided on a show and are firmly committed to competing, you will need to fill out the entry form. Most entry forms are available for download on the show information site or promoter's site. These forms are a wealth of information and will tell you just about everything you need to know regarding the competition including: classes, fees, locations, times, rules, and awards. It's a good idea to print of an extra form so you can have all the information handy.

Classes:

Within each major class (Bikini, Figure, Fitness, Physique, and Bodybuilding) are subcategories in which you will need to decide where to compete. The subcategories include: Masters, Beginner, Novice, Open, and Wheelchair. To subcategorize even further, these are usually broken down into age (Masters only), height, and weight. Depending on the promoter, Federation, and number of competitors, this can vary from show to show.

Masters:

Most Federations consider 35 to be the qualifying age

to compete in the Master category. Again, depending on the show promoter, there can be numerous age categories to further separate the classes out such as 35-39, 40-49, 50-59, and so on. If there is a large amount of competitors within one category, it will most likely be broken down even further into a classification system of A, B, C, D, etc. For example, if you are eligible to compete in the 35-39 Figure Master division and there are 20 other girls who will also be competing in that division, chances are, the promoter will further separate you out based on height and you will now be in a more specific group of 35-39 Figure Master, Class B. If on the other hand, there are only 5 women competing in that particular age category, the promoter could opt to have only the one class, thus making you all compete in one grouping.

Teen:

This category is usually only seen in the Bodybuilding class. You must be a teenager between the ages of 13-19 by a certain date. A specific cut off birth date will also be listed. If the entry form says you must be between the ages of 13-19 on July 15th, you would still be eligible to compete in this class even if you turn 20 years old on July 16th. Just make sure you are aware of the time frame you are given.

Collegiate:

Not all shows have this category, but occasionally can come across a competition with this option. As with the Teen category, this is usually limited to bodybuilding. To qualify for this class, you must be a college student. Be prepared to show a college identification card at the time of check in.

Beginner:

Some shows offer this category and some don't. You will need to verify via the entry form or promoter if this is an option. A beginner category is usually limited to first time competitors who have never competed before. Depending on the Federation and class you are in, this can be broken down even further by height or weight.

Novice:

You can qualify for Novice if you have competed before, but have not won your category. I'm not sure anyone actually confirms your eligibility for this category, but it is highly frowned upon if you really shouldn't be competing in this category yet enter it anyway. This is a great category for first time competitors as well as those who do not have much experience. Although you are not eligible to win your pro card in this category, they do still award an overall winner. As with the other categories, this can be broken down into further subcategories by height or weight.

Open:

The open category is the melting pot of all the other categories. Anyone is eligible to compete in this category no matter past competition placements, age, or experience. This is the most "popular" class to enter, especially among those competitors who are seeking out their Pro card. It is the only category that is eligible for pro status. Remember, within the NPC you are only eligible for Pro status if you are competing in a National level show. It is important to note that some shows will have the winner(s) of the Master Division included in the lineup for the overall judging. If the winner of the Master division wins the overall against the other open winners, then she will win her Pro card (if the show is awarding Pro cards).

Wheelchair:

This category is open to anyone who is in a wheelchair, and is usually prevalent in bodybuilding. If you have a disability, but are not confined to a wheelchair, you are NOT eligible for this category. Depending on the number of competitors, this category can also be broken down by age and/or competition experience.

Height vs. Weight:

It is not an accident that I have not specified specifically if a category is subcategorized by weight or height. If you are competing in a tested show, chances are you will be divided by height, even if you are a bodybuilder. If you are competing in a non-tested show, there is a good likelihood you will be divided up within your category based on your weight. The entry form will explain how you will be divided up, right down to the ½ pound or ¼" and you will be asked to mark which subcategory you believe you will compete in. They will verify your appropriate category during check in.

I should add that this is only applicable to bodybuilders. If you are competing in any of the other categories, you will most definitely be placed by height.

How many categories can I enter?

You can compete in as many categories that you are eligible for. It is plausible for you to meet all requirements to compete in Novice, Masters, and Open. I'm a firm believer in competing in anything you are eligible for, after all, you have spent months getting ready, and a decent amount of money in the process; you might as well walk away with a few awards if possible! Just remember, there is usually one entry fee for the first class and then a discounted entry fee PER each additional class you compete in, so keep that in mind when deciding.

What does it mean to "cross- over"?

If you decide to compete in two completely different, major, categories you are doing what they call, "Crossing Over." For example, if you are going to enter as a Bikini competitor, but also want to try your hand at Figure, you can certainly compete as both and cross over between Bikini and Figure. There are usually set rules about how many categories you can cross between, and some are even more specific saying you can't cross over between specific classes. Check the rules on the entry form to verify they allow this; as I've seen some shows prohibit any crossing over at all. Just as above, be prepared to pay for every category you are competing in.

Fees:

Not only will you have fees associated with the number of categories you will be entering, but you will also be required to purchase a membership in the Federation you are going to be competing in. The cost to join the Federation varies depending on which one it is. Once you purchase your membership, you will be able to compete in any shows, within that Federation, for a year. Take note on whether the membership is good for a full year, or if it expires at the end of the calendar year.

IMPORTANT: You will not be allowed to compete in the show if you are not a member. Most Federations allow the membership to be purchased during check in, however, if uncertain you can always request it by mail. If using the mail system, allow PLENTY of time to receive your card or else you will not have proof of your membership come show time.

Polygraph:

If you are participating in a tested show, depending on which Federation you are competing in, you will be required to take a polygraph prior to the show. Once the promoter has received your entry form, they will schedule a polygraph date and time which you will be required to attend. During the test, you will be asked a series of questions regarding the use of banned substances. If you do not pass the test, you will not be allowed to compete in the show. It is my understanding that any questionable results will be discussed with the promoter, allowing them to decide if you should be able to compete or not. Currently, the competitor is responsible for paying for this test and required to submit payment at the time of service.

Tickets:

The entry form will also provide information regarding the purchase of tickets for the event. Sometimes the entry form includes a section for you to buy the tickets; whereas other times it will provide information as to where they can be purchased. Usually the ticket buying options are broken down into: pre-judging (open seating), finals (VIP and assigned seating), or a combo, allowing you to purchase morning and evening shows at a discounted price. Some of the larger shows sell out very quickly, so be diligent in purchasing your tickets in advance to ensure good seating.

Closing thoughts:

If you are on a tight budget, you can easily spread these costs out over a short period of time. Also be sure to allow plenty of time to submit your entry form in order to avoid having to pay a late fee. Just remember, almost every cost associated with entering the show is non-refundable, so be sure of your commitment before you start paying for things.

Location:

The entry form will be a wealth of information regarding where and when the events will take place. Although sometimes check in, tanning, and the show itself are all in one place, more often than not, they take place at different locations. Be sure you are certain of where you are expected to be and at what time, to avoid being left out of the show. If you are not familiar with the area you are competing in, it would be a good idea to locate the different places prior to the time you are required to be there.

Rules:

As stated before, the rules regarding the show will be found on the entry form. You will be able to see what is allowed, and what is prohibited. Make sure you familiarize yourself with these rules, as they are listed for a specific reason. Right now, the NPC does not allow the use Dream Tan (a tanning product). If you show up wearing Dream Tan, you will most likely be prohibited from competing or be required to shower it off.

There will also be rules regarding length of music (Fitness, Physique, Bodybuilding), who will perform their routine, suits, jewelry, and so on. The Federations are usually pretty strict on making sure their rules are abided by. Again, each Federation has a set of rules and could differ from show to show. Everything you need to know regarding what is accepted or prohibited is clearly listed on the entry form. If you have any questions, contact the promoter for clarification.

Awards:

The best part of the whole show…the awards. These can vary greatly between shows and Federations. The entry form will not only tell you which placements will be given awards, but will tell you exactly what the awards consist of. I've seen trophies include: statues, goblets, medals, swords, crystals, platters, and crystal bowls. Check the entry form for details.

Chapter 10
Traveling

Almost every show has a designated hotel, or host hotel, for the competitors to stay at. Promoters have usually chosen the hotel based on its location to the venue and have negotiated a lower rate by reserving a large number of rooms. Usually, other services such as tanning, makeup, and registration are also done in the host hotel out of convenience to the competitors. Be certain to check the entry form for details regarding this though, as sometimes they are done at a different location. If you are planning on using the host hotel, be sure to book your room well in advance as almost all other out of town competitors will also be utilizing this service.

It is not a requirement to stay at the host hotel. If you want to do a little research on surrounding hotels in order to do a price comparison, then that is perfectly acceptable. No matter where you end up staying, be sure to note the hotel amenities. Although most hotels offer similar things, you will want to confirm the availability of a microwave and a refrigerator. Remember, you will be taking enough food to get you through 2-3 days, so having those two amenities is a must!

Competing outside of your hometown is definitely a little more stressful and requires more attention to details. If you are 400 miles away from home and realize your shoes have been left on the bed, you could be in a serious predicament. If planning on competing out of town, be sure to allow plenty of time to get a list together of things required for your competition. If you are flying, I highly suggest you take a carry-on bag containing everything you need to step on stage that way if your regular bag gets lost you will still be able to compete.

With that being said, let's discuss some points to consider when traveling out of town and some items you will want to make sure go with you.

How long to get there?

Whether or not you are flying or driving out of town, you need to allow plenty of time for travel and arrival. Check-in is usually the night before the show, and is restricted to a specific time frame. Be sure your departure and arrival time correspond with the times designated for hotel check-in, tanning, and competition check-in.

Date of departure/return:

Most people arrive in their destination city the day prior

to the show, and leave the morning after the show. As long as you allow yourself plenty of time to attend the required check-ins and meetings, the arrival time is up to you. Just be sure to allow yourself plenty of time to get checked into the hotel and familiar with the designated locations prior to the time you need to be there.

Although it is common to leave the morning after the competition, be sure to note any rules regarding this. Some shows (especially at the National level) require the winners of certain classes to attend a mandatory photo shoot the next morning. If you drove to the show, this is usually not a big problem. However, if you booked a flight to leave the next morning thus interfering with your availability to attend the photo shoot, this could pose a big problem. If a promoter specifically states the requirement to attend the photo shoot, they mean business. If this happens, you should be prepared to change the time of your departing flight and expect to pay any fees associated with the change.

Items to pack:

- Enough food to get you through your competition
- Water
- Measuring cups/food scale

- Containers for food
- Utensils
- Map/directions to hotel (if needed)
- Hotel confirmation number
- Hotel information (address, phone number)
- Cash/checks/debit card/credit card
- Sheets (hotels will charge a fee if you stain their sheets with tanning solution)
- Extra towels (fee applies to stained hotel towels as well)
- Two suitcases (main suitcase and competition suitcase)
- Shampoo, conditioner, hair products
- Food cooler
- Ice packs
- Competition shoes (if applicable)
- Suit(s)
- Competition makeup
- Fake eyelashes (if applicable)
- Competition jewelry
- Brush/comb
- Curling iron/flat iron
- Phone and charger
- Show information

- Camera/charger
- Pam/glaze
- Inserts for suit (if applicable)
- Suit glue/tape
- Razor (new)
- Bobby pins, hair clips, barrettes
- Baby wipes (to wipe face/hands after tan has been applied)
- Hairspray
- Needle/thread/safety pins (to fix suit in case of mishap)
- Scissors (if you haven't cut your straps to fit you)
- ID (driver's license)
- Organization membership card (if already purchased)
- Pump up bands (optional)
- Cotton swabs
- Cover up(you will need to wear loose, oversized clothing after you have been tanned. I suggest going to thrift store and purchasing a pair of scrubs and a men's large button down top)
- Flip flops or sandals (no tennis shoes after tan is applied)
- IPod, book, or some form of entertainment to

keep you busy while waiting to be called to stage.

This is a just a general idea of items you will want to have with you. Again, allow yourself a good week or two to compile your own list, and to allow plenty of time to get things purchased and packed. To save some time, you can pack all competition items into your separate comp bag before you travel, and if possible, take as a carry on if flying.

Chapter 11
The day before competition!

The day before your competition will be filled with nerves and a lot of running around! Registration, check-in and tanning are just a few of the things you will be required to attend within the day and early evening. The entry form will always have the location and times of the registration, so be sure to familiarize yourself with all the details. If you are utilizing the show tanning service, you should have also received a scheduled time in which you will need to arrive. Note that sometimes the tanning service is in a different location from the check-in. Depending on the timing of events, you will need to know if you will be attending registration or tanning first and allow ample time for both.

Tanning:

Although we discussed tanning a little in previous chapters, it is important to get an idea of some of the details associated with this process. If you are under the impression that you will simply show up, get sprayed, and leave, you will probably be surprised at how much preparation is required. As touched upon before, almost all tanning companies will provide you with a list of preparations you will need to complete before getting your tan applied.

- Shaving: the tanning solution applied to your body will adhere to any hair that is present. With this being said, you will need to shave every inch of your body from your neck down to your toes. The best way to do this is to purchase a brand new razor, a good shaving cream, and enlist the help of someone you feel comfortable with. (A full length mirror is also a consideration). Most tanning companies ask that you shave the day/night PRIOR to having your tan applied. If you are scheduled to be tanned on Friday, it would be best to shave Thursday evening. This allows the pores plenty of time to close up, and avoids any tanning solution seeping into them, thus creating a speckled look. Remember, your WHOLE body needs to be shaved, including your back, buttocks, chest, arms etc.

- Exfoliate: it is usually a good idea to start exfoliating your body daily, approximately one week before show time. This removes any dry skin from your body, allowing for a smooth looking tan. Any dry patches on your skin will absorb more tanning solution and could leave you looking blotchy. Do not underestimate the importance of this step and be sure to include your back in the process.

- No lotions/deodorant: be sure you do not have any lotion, face cream, sprays, or deodorant on your skin immediately prior to having your tan applied. Any product on your skin will have a reaction to the solution, thus turning your skin a greenish color. This is not an appealing look and will cause undue stress, so be sure your skin is clean and free of lotions/creams.

- Wash hair/shower: once your tan is applied you will not be allowed to shower. If you shave on Thursday evening, you are free to shower one last time on Friday, prior to your tanning appointment. This is the time you will want to make sure your hair is washed, as you will most likely not be able to wash it again until the competition is over. Be sure to take a shower cap with you to the tanning appointment, if they do not provide one.

- Cover up: once your tan is applied, you will not be allowed to wear tight fitting clothes of any sort. If you do not have any clothing you are willing to stain, I highly suggest going to a local thrift store and purchasing a large pair of scrub pants, and an oversized button down shirt to wear afterwards. I favor button down shirts to avoid having to pull a shirt off over my head; thus taking the chance of messing up my hair or makeup once I start prepping for the show.

- Flip flops: your feet will also be tanned and you will be advised to wear sandals or flip flops in lieu of tennis shoes and or socks. These do not have to be anything fancy, and can be purchased fairly cheap if you don't want to chance staining a good pair.

As always, be sure to follow all suggested procedures the tanning company provides. They are professionals and know what will ensure the best looking tan. Although some of the details can seem a bit monotonous or tedious, do not skip them as they can make the difference between a great looking tan and a disaster.

Registration/check-in:

The registration/check-in is a first come first serve basis. All competitors are required to attend the check-in or they will not be allowed to compete. With that being said, you can certainly surmise this could be a very lengthy process if you are competing in a large show with a few hundred competitors. If you have scheduled your tanning AFTER you check -in, be sure to allow approximately 1-1.5 hours to complete registration. If you have never competed before, here are some things you can expect to happen at registration and some tips to help you get through the process as smoothly as possible.

Let me add one huge piece of advice here that I'm sure you will NOT adhere to: keep your eyes to yourself! I am also incapable of following this piece of advice, even though over the years I have finally started learning my lesson. Listen, every single competitor is going to be there, including girls who will be in your class. It is human nature to look around and kind of "check out" the competition. The problem with this is that you have no clue if the girl you are freaking out about is actually YOUR competition or not. I've been known to go into a major panic over a girl who was leaner than I was, had fuller muscles etc. only to find out she was a Bodybuilder and NOT a Figure competitor. Plus, there are so many things you CAN'T see, like how tight their butt is, how they perform on stage, and what their overall package consists of. So, although I KNOW you are going to scope everyone out and compare yourself to them, keep in mind that you have no way of knowing if this person is a "threat" or not.

Federation Membership:

If you opted to purchase your membership at the check-in, this is where you will get it. Before you are allowed to complete any other part of your registration process, you will need to purchase the membership. Be sure to have a check or cash with you. After filling out the membership card with your personal information and submitting payment, you will be given a receipt. Make sure you hold on to the receipt and keep it in a safe place. If you are competing in a future show, and haven't received your permanent card in the mail, you will need to show proof of purchase in order to compete in the next competition. If you forget to take it with you, you will be required to purchase another membership.

Height:

If you are competing in Bikini, Figure, Fitness, Women's Physique, or (sometimes) Bodybuilding, you will be asked to stand against a wall, barefoot, so your height can be confirmed. Some of the classes are divided by as little as ¼" so they are very careful to confirm your height in order to place you in the correct height class. The bodybuilding class can be divided by either height or weight, depending on the organization in which you are competing.

(If you are curious as to how many girls are in your class, this is the time to inquire. Just be aware that the girls listed on the check in sheet in your class are based on the information entered on the entry form, and could change if they misrepresented their height. This number can change either way once heights are confirmed.)

Weight:

If you are participating in a show that classifies bodybuilders by weight, you will be asked to strip down to your posing suit. You will then be weighed and categorized accordingly. You are not allowed to wear any other clothing except a posing suit for weigh in.

Suit Check:

All organizations have very strict rules on what is considered appropriate regarding the cut of your suit. The main restriction being that it CANNOT be a thong, or even closely resemble one. A quick suit check is usually required during the time you are height checked or weighed. It is not usually required to be wearing your suit during this time unless you are a bodybuilder being weighed. Just make sure and take your suit to registration should you be asked to show that it meets their requirements.

Age:

If you are competing in a category that is classified by age, be prepared to show proof. I've never been asked to verify my age, but the entry form does clearly state to bring an ID of some sort (driver's license or birth certificate) for confirmation should you be asked. It's always best to be prepared and have your ID handy even if you don't think you have any reason to take it.

Music:

If you are competing in Fitness, Physique, or Bodybuilding you will be required to do a routine. Again, be sure to check the entry form for timing restrictions in regards to the length of your music. It is NEVER acceptable to perform to a song that contains profanity, and usually ends in a disqualification. Be sure to have your CD clearly labeled with your first and last name, and the category in which you are competing. Promoters usually ask for a copy of your music during check-in so be sure to have it ready. It is always wise to have a back-up copy on hand in case of some unforeseen event.

DVD's:

There is usually a person hired to videotape the whole show. This does not apply to all shows, but is becoming prevalent. If a videographer has been hired, there is a good chance they will have an area set up where you can purchase DVD's of the show. Most offer three options: prejudging only, night show only, or both (usually at a discounted rate). There is no requirement to purchase, but make great presents for family members who weren't able to attend. If you think you might want to purchase a DVD of your competition, make sure and take some sort of payment. Although it's usually possible to purchase the DVD's at a later date, ones that are purchased PRIOR to the show are usually discounted.

Final thoughts:

After you have completed check-in and tanning, it is important to try to relax as much as possible. Being on your feet for an extended amount of time (especially in the heat) can cause exhaustion and swelling. Too much running around can also encourage sweating, which will make your tan run. Although you are going to be excited, try to use the rest of your evening to relax, double check items that need to be packed in your competition bag, set your alarm, make sure your phone/camera are charged, and tend to last minute details. Once everything is squared away for the evening, try getting some sleep (easier said than done); tomorrow is going to be a long and exhausting day!!

Chapter 12

Competition Day!

All the months of training, dieting, posing practice, stressing, and obsessing have brought you to this day. Although at the time, it seemed as if the competition would never get here, you are most likely now in shock that the time has actually come for you to showcase all your hard work, dedication, and sacrifice. Take a deep breath and take this moment in… let's go!

Prep:

Make sure you have allowed plenty of time to complete all prep needed. If you are not used to applying fake eyelashes, believe me, this can be a good hour long process. Although you will most likely have plenty of time for touch-up's at the competition, it is wise to be as "put together" ahead of time as you can, so you aren't pressured for time at the show.

When it comes to wearing your suit to the competition, that micro decision is up to you. Once you get your suit on, it is best to avoid taking it off and on numerous times, for fear of messing up the tan. If you would prefer taking the suit with you to the venue and changing into it once you arrive, that is also perfectly acceptable. Just make sure, as with everything else, you allow plenty of time to get changed. Sometimes the shows run very quickly (especially if a smaller show), and your backstage time is very limited. If in doubt, your best bet is to wear the suit to the show and then just adjust it once backstage. Remember, the goal is to be as prepared as possible; don't save a lot of "last minute things" for the show.

Pack Food Bag:

You will most certainly be required to eat specific foods, set forth by your trainer, throughout your wait to get on stage and prejudging. Make sure you have your cooler packed with all food (plus more) required to get you through the morning show. I added "plus more" in here due to the fact some shows run much later than anticipated. The last thing you want to deal with is not having adequate amounts of food with you in case this scenario should arise. Also be sure you have packed any utensils needed, as well as wet wipes or napkins. It is strongly advised to take your food in a separate bag from your competition bag to avoid damaging shoes, suits, makeup etc. in case of spillage.

Competition Bag:

This was touched on a few times in earlier chapters. Anything and everything you will need to help you in regards to backstage prep needs to be included in this bag. Some must haves are: competition makeup, hair spray, curling iron/straight iron, shoes, back up cd, brush, needle/thread, safety pins, hand towel, Pam spray, back up suit (if taking one), suit glue, Q-tips, baby wipes, membership card, ID, warm up bands, and nails/nail glue (if wearing press on). If in doubt, TAKE IT!!

Competitor Meeting:

All competitors will be required to attend the competitor meeting, a few hours prior to the start of the competition. The meeting is almost always held in the exact same location as where the actual show and judging will take place. During this time, you will be given your competitor number, introduced to the judges, given a run-down of how the show will be organized, shown mandatory poses and the correct way to perform them, and then allowed to ask questions. During this meeting you will learn everything you need to know regarding the competition, including the rules, location of prep rooms, and order of events. Be sure to ask for clarification on anything you might have questions about.

More prepping/final touches:

The competitor meeting usually ends just a few minutes prior to the start of pre-judging. Once the meeting is over, you will want to locate the room designated for changing and prepping. If you are among the first group to be on stage, you will want to be sure to locate this room immediately and start putting all finishing touches on your prep. If your tan got smeared or disturbed in any way, you will need to get in line for touch up's immediately. Unlike the first time you were tanned, you will need to wear your suit for touch-ups. This is also the time you will need to make sure your suit is fitted to you, glued or taped in place if needed, and your glaze (or Pam) applied.

Pump up:

All shows have a designated coordinator to keep all competitors a breast to the next group headed to stage for judging. Usually they will walk around backstage, and say something like, "Master Figure, Class A, you are up in about 15 minutes." Once you hear this, you will need to start pumping up. There is always a designated pump up area, loaded with free weights and bands (use your bands to ensure having access to weights) you can use. Most competitors begin high repetition movements with light weights, in order to fill the muscle with blood and create a pump. This gives the illusion of full, hard muscles when on stage; which is usually the effect most competitors are trying to achieve. Be sure you allow time to pump up, just be cautious not to do this too far out from the time you will be on stage.

Line up:

When the group before you is on the stage, the coordinator will most likely start lining the next class up. Once you know your group will be on stage shortly, it is imperative to stay around the coordinator in order to be present when he calls for line up. Most of them make it more than clear, during the competitor meeting, that they will only call your number a limited amount of time for line up. If you are not present and do not make it into the line with the rest of your class, you will be marked off the judging sheet and not allowed to compete in that class. Be certain to listen for your number, and acknowledge the coordinator when they call for you. You will be lined up in numerical order and then asked to wait until it is time to hit the stage.

Stage time:

Depending on the show, how you enter the stage can vary greatly. Sometimes you are asked to enter one at a time, go center stage, perform a couple poses, and then wait on the side of the stage for other girls in your class to do the same thing. Once all girls have completed their poses and are on stage, you will all be filed in a single line to the center of the stage for judging to begin. Some shows will have you enter the stage at the same time as the other competitors in your group, and symmetry judging begins immediately. The free style posing (sometimes called the T-walk) is then done after symmetry judging is complete, whereas sometimes it is not done at all. Due to the increasing numbers of competitors, most organizations are cutting the T-walk, and opting for a couple free style poses to be done just prior to symmetry. Again, all this will be discussed at the morning meeting and reiterated just prior to approaching the stage.

Large groups:

If your group has a minimum amount of girls, it is most likely you will all be judged at one time and placed ac-

cordingly before being asked to leave the stage. However, if your category has a large number of competitors in it, the judges will usually split it into two or three
smaller groups. Most of the time, all the competitors
will be brought to center stage in single file line and
asked to complete a full round of quarter turns. During
this time, the judges get an overall idea of the total
package each person is presenting and can start nar-
rowing the group down to the top contenders. Once
you have performed one to two full rounds of symmetry
comparisons, the judges will ask you to return to the
side of the stage you were at, in the order you were
brought out.

First call out:

Once the first round of symmetry is complete and all
competitors have returned to their original place on the
side of the stage, the head judge will announce a first
call out, asking certain numbers to come back to the
center of the stage. It is no secret that making the first
call out is every girl's goal. The girls called back to the
stage during this time, are 99% guaranteed a top five
spot in the placements. The girls called back out, will
be compared against each other in all aspects (symmetry, mandatory poses, overall look, stage presence
etc.) and placed accordingly. After they have been
placed, they will be asked to return to their original
place on the side of the stage and a second call out
will take place, and placements 6th- whatever will be

determined. In very large shows, like a National level show, it is not uncommon for there to be six or more total call outs.

The bubble:

If you notice, I said the girls in first call out are usually 99% certain to be top five. If the competition between girls is very tough, it is possible to be on "the bubble" in your placement. Here is an example of how this works: if you are among the first five called out, and look to be in consideration for 4th or 5th place, they might ask the girls, who they know placed top three, to go back to the side of the stage, leaving two girls from the first call out still on stage. The judges will then announce the second call out and ask those girls to join the two remaining on stage. If you end up in the center spot among this group, you are pretty much guaranteed the 4th place finish. However, the two girls (usually one on each side of center person) who are most likely in contention for 5th place are not guaranteed the spot. If you are the person who is either going to win 5th or 6th, you care considered to be "on the bubble," meaning you might not know your placement until finals.

Placements:

There is a good rule of thumb when trying to determine how you placed within your category. If you were among the first call out, and asked to move to the center of the stage, you can USUALLY consider yourself the winner. Girls get asked to move around all the time during comparisons. The head judge usually makes sure the winner of the group is positioned in the center (most stages have an X on them to indicate center), with the 2nd and 3rd place finisher on each side of her. Once a general idea of placements is achieved, you will be asked to perform more symmetry rounds and/or mandatories. If during this time the judges notice a competitor is not placed correctly, they will ask that competitor to change spots with someone else within the group. Once all placements have been decided and judging is over, the judge will thank you, and the group will be asked to exit the stage.

*IMPORTANT NOTE: Remember, you are also being judged on stage presence at all time. Even when you are switching places with someone else, be sure you are SMILING and working your stage presence angle! When you are walking or standing on the side of the stage you are still being judged! A good rule of thumb is, if you are on stage (no matter where you are standing) you are being judged, so make sure you display yourself in the appropriate manner! I've seen a smile (vs. a girl who didn't smile) be the "tie breaker" in a really tight placement. (True story)

Scoring:

Each judge is provided with a list of all the competitors within each class. As you are asked to perform your symmetry and mandatory poses, the judges will begin placing/ranking you on their score sheet. Your goal is to have as many judges as possible give you a ranking of "1" or first place. After all judges have decided the placements, they will hand the score sheets down to a score keeper. The score keeper will then make off the highest and lowest score, per competitor, and add up the remaining scores. If for instance, six judges gave you a placement of first, and one judge gave you a placement of second, one of the first place scores, and the second place score would be crossed off and the remaining five scores of first place would be added up to give you a total of "5" for your final score. The goal is to get the lowest score of all the competitors, as this means you have earned a first place. The competitor with the next lowest score will then be awarded second, and so on.

Multiple Classes:

If you are only competing in one class, you are free to leave until the night show. If you are in more than one class or category, be sure to stay fairly close to the co-ordinator in order to hear when you will be required to line up again. If you are in Master Figure and Figure Open Class A, it is most likely you will be required to line up immediately for Open, after finishing your Master class pre-judging. Being aware of the order of events and listening closely to the coordinator will ensure a smooth transition between each category. If you are competing in two separate categories completely (Figure and Physique), it is possible to experience a huge gap in time before required to step back on stage. This is when some sort of entertainment comes in handy. You can also opt to go watch the other classes being judged, just be sure to wear your cover up, and try your best to take it easy. Just allow plenty of time for any touch up's you might need to do, and make sure you are accessible backstage prior to your class being called.

End of Pre-Judging:

Once you have been judged in all classes and categories you entered, you are free to leave the venue. This is the time when most competitors head back home (or hotel) to relax, eat, and update family/friends of the morning's happenings. Although you will most likely be running on adrenaline from the morning judging (especially if you feel you did really well), it is important to take it as easy as you can because the night show usually lasts late into the evening. If prejudging ended late, you might not have much time to do anything before needing to be back for finals. If this is the case, it is best to go somewhere close to grab a bite to eat or just sit with family and friends. Make sure you are aware of the time you are required to be back at the venue for the evening meeting, and allow ample time to ensure you arrive on time.

Chapter 13

Finals

The night show, or finals, is run completely different than pre-judging and is considered more of a production. Once you arrive back at the venue for the competitors evening meeting, you will most certainly notice all the awards lined up on a table on stage, promoters and judges wearing dressy clothing, the MC practicing his/her speech, colorful stage lighting, music, and maybe even a professional guest poser somewhere in the wings. During the meeting, you will be informed of any updates to the show, the order of events, routines, and all relevant information regarding the award process, structure and so forth.

Updates:

Sometimes after pre-judging, the judges decide to change an aspect of the show. I've been involved in a competition that originally stated that the overall winner of a show was awarded their Pro card. After pre-judging, the head judge of the Pro organization decided the winner of each height category would be awarded their Pro card, and not limited to the overall. There is also a possibility that during calculation of the scores, a tie was discovered. If this is the case, the judges will announce a comparison judging among the girls involved in the tie, or an alternate plan of action to decide the class. All information regarding anything like this will be addressed during the evening meeting.

Order of events:

Although the evening show almost always runs in the same order as pre-judging, there are always extra events added in. Most shows have hired a guest poser to attend the event to provide further entertainment to the crowd. The promoters will have a complete run down of the order of events as well as how the show will be run in regards to introducing competitors, routines, awards, pictures, and overall comparisons.

Introducing competitors: Unlike the morning show, all competitors will be brought on to the stage individually. During this time, the MC will read from a card you filled out (either on entry form or at a meeting) stating any personal information or "thank you" acknowledgements you wrote down. While the MC is reading your information, you will most likely be performing a t-walk or random poses of your choice. The poses vs. t-walk varies between shows, the promoter will inform you of the correct procedure. After completing your stage time, you will then be asked to exit the stage.

Once you exit the stage, the coordinator will ask you to "hang out" backstage while waiting for the other girls in your class to be introduced. After they have all gotten through their introductions and made their way off stage, the MC will announce the top five (in no particular order), and ask them to come back out to the stage.

Sometimes, as you exit the stage, the coordinator will immediately tell you if you secured a top five spot and request that you stay close by. If you have not secured a top five spot, you are free to leave the area (or go home if not involved in any other classes) until your next category is up.

If competing in multiple classes, you will only be "formally" introduced one time. During subsequent classes you are involved in, the MC will simply state your name and make it known that you have already been introduced, but are also competing in the current category. Most likely you will not be required to go back on stage for introductions; however will need to stay close by until the top five are announced.

Routines: Fitness, Physique, and Bodybuilder competitors will complete a routine as part of the evening show. (Fitness also performs their routine during pre-judging which accounts for 1/3 of their total score)Depending on the size of the show, and at the discrepancy of the promoter, not everyone will be allowed to perform their routine. It is not uncommon for routines to be performed only by the competitors who have secured a top five placement. However, there are many shows who allow EVERY competitor, whether they place or not, the opportunity to perform their routine. While the MC is reading your bio, you will most likely be waiting center stage to begin your routine. Some girls choose to wait off stage while bio is being read, while others enter the stage and stand in their beginning position until it is time to begin their routine.

Awards:

If you have secured a top five spot and are called back on to stage, you will simply walk on stage and stand in a single line next to the other four top finishers. You will most likely notice the X that once marked center stage has now been replaced with the numbers one through five. Once all girls are back on stage, the MC will begin announcing the placements, starting with 5th place. If you hear your number/name called, simply raise your hand to acknowledge the placement. Once the award has been placed in your hand (or around your neck) the person who handed you the award will direct you to move to the number on the stage, which corresponds with your placement. After all placements and awards have been announced, competitors will be asked to pose for a group picture. More often than not, the winner of the class will be asked to stay on stage, while the other top four competitors exit, for a "winners" photo. Afterwards, be certain to show gratitude to the judges and audience for your placement, and exit the stage.

Overall Comparison:

Some categories offer an Overall winner. The overall winner is considered the winner of the whole show within that category. How this works is that the winner of each individual class (we will use Figure in this case), will be asked to return to the stage once all classes within the Figure category have been announced. If there were four classes (A, B, C, D and sometimes Masters is included in the overall comparison), the winners of each class will come back on to stage and be compared to the other winners. The judges will follow the exact same judging procedures as they did for pre-judging. Each winner will be compared on symmetry, muscle, tone, stage presence, and so forth. If any girls need to be moved, the judges will call out the numbers that need to switch places. Once each judge has decided who they believe has won, they will write the competitor's number on a piece of paper and hand it to the head judge. The head judge will tally up the votes and then give the number of the overall winner to the MC. The MC will announce who has won the Overall, and that competitor will be given additional awards.

Overall Tie:

It is possible for the judges to be split when it comes to deciding an overall winner. If the score is tied, it is typical procedure for the head judge to make the tie breaking decision. They will usually announce that a tie has occurred and then leave it in the hands of the head judge to make the final vote. It is possible to be asked to do another round of symmetry in order to help with the decision. Make sure you are always "on" and assume you are being judged at all times, until the final decision has been decided. As with the other categories, be prepared to pose for an overall picture as well as a winner picture.

Pro card:

As stated in previous chapters, it is possible to earn a pro card based on how you place in the competition. Usually, Pro status is awarded to the overall winner within each category. If you have won the overall in your category, in a show that is a Pro Qualifier, you will now be considered a Pro competitor within that organization. Depending on the procedure, your pro card will either be mailed to you, or you will be given a form to fill out requesting your pro card. If you have achieved pro status, you are now eligible to compete in "Professional" competitions against other Pro's. Awards on this level more often than not, include a monetary prize along with the award.

Urine Test:

If you have entered a tested show, and have placed within the top five in your category, you will be required to submit urine for a drug test. It is extremely important you give a urine sample before leaving the show. If you leave the competition without performing the test, you will be disqualified and forfeit your award and placement. Usually the coordinator of the show (or promoter) will whisk you to the nearest bathroom right as you walk off stage. Be prepared; the urine test is an "open door" test. This means the bathroom door will have to remain open while you pee into the cup just to make sure there is no way to compromise the sample. After you hand your sample over, an information sheet will be filled out and a sticker will be placed on your sample cup for identification. IF you fail the drug screening, you will be prohibited from participating in that organization for approximately seven years, your award and placement will be taken away, and the competitor who received 2nd, will now be considered the 1st place winner.

Nationally Qualified:

If you have competed in a show labeled as a "National Qualifier" and have placed accordingly (sometimes this is limited to top three in each class, other times it is limited to the first place winner or overall) you are now qualified to compete in a National level show. These competitions consist only of other competitors who have qualified via their placement within a national qualifying event. Within the NPC, you must win or earn a specific placement at a national show in order to be awarded Professional status.

Post show:

After the entire show has concluded, many competitors and judges go to a "host" restaurant for a little post show gathering. The restaurant is usually close to the venue and has been secured for the competitor gathering. Most establishments have agreed to stay open later than normal as well as offer deals to the participants of the show. Although this is not a required event, it is usually a lot of fun to be able to hang with fellow competitors and perhaps get feedback from the judges.

Washing your suit:

After all the festivities of the night are over and you have made it back home, you will certainly want to shower (you won't believe how good this shower is going to feel!!) to get the excess tan and glaze off of your body. If possible, you will need to plan on washing your suit within the next day. Although most girls are a little scared of washing their suit, it is actually a very easy process.

- Rinse your suit under warm running water.
- Fill sink with warm water.
- Put a small amount of laundry detergent on a fingernail brush and LIGHTLY scrub at any area that needs extra attention. DO NOT scrub the outside of your suit as it can damage the material and stones.
- Immerse suit into sink a few times to get the soap out. Agitate the suit back and forth to work some of the tanning solution out, but DO NOT soak the suit as it will cause the stones to come off of the material.
- Once you are finished cleaning suit, empty sink, carefully wring the suit out with your hands, and lay the suit flat on a towel to dry.

- After suit has dried, it can now be stored in a large zip lock bag until it is needed again.

Chapter 14

Post Competition Eating disorders/Body Image Disorders and Depression

After many months of low calories, food restrictions, excessive workouts, and extreme focus on your competition, you are now told to, "Enjoy your offseason." While most competitors are thrilled with the idea of being able to eat all once forbidden food when and where they want it, that excitement can be very short lived. After months of structure and watching your physique transform into a competitor state, it can be quite shocking to see what effect all the goodies you are consuming can have on your body, and within a relatively short amount of time. If you are not prepared for this fast and often negatively perceived change, you could be faced with quite a shock. Many girls are not prepared, mentally, for the weight gain and immediate changes that happen to their body once they start eating anything other than a competition diet and thus become filled with anxiety that can lead to depression, eating disorders, and body image disorders.

Eating disorders, body image disorders, and depression are very real and serious problems which can be magnified or even caused by the competition process. As discussed in a previous chapter, it is not uncommon for friends and family to become concerned with your extremely low body fat and wonder if you are suffering from some sort of disorder. Although some girls are very much aware of a previous struggle with a disorder or depression prior to competing, others do not realize they have developed one, until after the competition is over and they struggle to find a balance with non-structured eating and their changing body.

On a personal note, I have struggled with anorexia and body image disorder for approximately 24 years. Admittedly, I saw that by entering a competition I could find a more "accepted" outlet for my sickness. After all, by obtaining single digit body fat percentage and eating the bare minimum my body required I could guarantee I would be "happy" with my physique and others would accept it as something required to be competitive in the sport.

During my years in the competition arena I have come across numerous girls, who like me, suffered with eating disorders and body image disorders and believed preparing for a show would serve as a way to control their symptoms or provide an outlet for their behavior. I've also come across quite a few who actually developed disorders and depression due to competing, and in the end confessed they wished they had never taken the competition path.

The fact that we take our body to such extremes can set the stage for unrealistic expectations of what we "should" look like. In fact, there has recently been a new body image disorder discovered called "Reverse Anorexia" and is prevalent in individuals who compete.

Let's take a closer look at a few of the main eating/body image disorders and discuss how they relate to competing.

Reverse Anorexia/Muscle Dysmorphia:

Wikipedia defines this disorder as follows: Muscle dysmorphia or bigorexia is a disorder in which a person becomes obsessed with the idea that they are not muscular enough. Those who suffer from muscle dysmorphia tend to hold delusions that they are "skinny" or "too small" but are often above average in musculature. Sometimes referred to as reverse anorexia nervosa, or the Adonis Complex, muscle dysmorphia is a very specific type of body dysmorphic disorder.

In this disorder a person is preoccupied with thoughts concerning appearance, especially musculature. Muscle dysmorphia is strictly connected with selective attention: individuals selectively focus their attention on perceived defect (too skinny body, underweight etc.). They are hyper vigilant to even small deviations from perceived ideal and they ignore information that their body image is not consistent with reality.

There is also a hypothesis that individuals repeat negative and distorted self-statements concerning their appearance to such extent that they become automatic. Muscle dysmorphia influences person's mood often causing depression or feelings of disgust. This is often connected with constant comparing of a person's body to unattainable ideal.

Muscle dysmorphia can cause people to:

- Constantly examine themselves in a mirror
- Frequently compare themselves with others
- Want to increase muscle mass
- Dream of lifting weights and exercise
- Become distressed if they miss a workout session or one of their many meals a day
- Become distressed if they do not receive enough protein per day in their   diet
- Use anabolic steroids, sometimes unsafely
- Neglect jobs, relationships, or family because of excessive exercising
- Have delusions of being underweight or below average in musculature.
- In extreme cases, inject appendages with fluid (e.g. synthol)
- Suffers from constant mood swings
- In extreme cases, being grumpy and short tempered

It is very easy to see how this disorder plays into the world of competing. In fact, it is mainly due to body-building that this disorder even came into existence. Although this disorder seems to be prevalent among male competitors, it can also be clearly seen within the female community of competitors as well. I admit I was never concerned with how much muscle mass I had until I began competing. I also noticed as I progressed into categories which required more muscle mass, I became more aware/obsessed with how much muscle I could gain, especially in my legs which I perceived to be the "weakest" of all body parts. If participating in a category which stresses muscle mass, beware that you could start experiencing this disorder.

Anorexia:

Wikipedia defines Anorexia as the following: Anorexia nervosa is an eating disorder characterized by immoderate food restriction and irrational fear of gaining weight, as well as a distorted body self-perception. It typically involves excessive weight loss. Anorexia nervosa usually develops during adolescence and early adulthood. Due to the fear of gaining weight, people with this disorder restrict the amount of food they consume. This restriction of food intake causes metabolic and hormonal disorders. Outside of medical literature, the terms anorexia nervosa and anorexia are often used interchangeably; however, anorexia is simply a medical term for lack of appetite and people with anorexia nervosa do not in fact, lose their appetites. Anorexia nervosa has many complicated implications and may be thought of as a lifelong illness that may never be truly cured, but only managed over time. Anorexia nervosa is characterized by low body weight, inappropriate eating habits and obsession with having a thin figure. Individuals suffering from it may also practice repetitive weighing, measuring, and mirror gazing, alongside other obsessive actions to make sure they are still thin, a common practice known as "body checking".

Anorexia nervosa is often coupled with a distorted self-image which may be maintained by various cognitive biases that alter how the affected individual evaluates and thinks about her or his body, food and eating. Anorexia nervosa is characterized by the fear of gaining weight. Those suffering from this disorder often view themselves as "too fat" even if they are already underweight. Persons with anorexia nervosa continue to feel hunger, but deny themselves all but very small quantities of food. The average caloric intake of a person with anorexia nervosa is 600–800 calories per day, but extreme cases of complete self-starvation are known. It is a serious mental illness with a high incidence of comorbidity and similarly high mortality rates to serious psychiatric disorders.

Between 50% and 75% of individuals with an eating disorder experience depression. In addition, 1 in 4 individuals who are diagnosed with anorexia nervosa also exhibit obsessive compulsive disorder.

Symptoms for a typical patient include:

- Refusal to maintain a normal body mass index for their age
- Amenorrhea, the absence of three consecutive menstrual cycles
- Fearful of even the slightest weight gain and takes all precautionary measures to avoid weight gain and becoming overweight
- Obvious, rapid, dramatic weight loss
- Lanugo: soft, fine hair growing on the face and body
- Obsession with calories and fat content of food
- Preoccupation with food, recipes, or cooking; may cook elaborate dinners for others, but not eat the food themselves
- Dieting despite being thin or dangerously underweight
- Rituals: cuts food into tiny pieces; refuses to eat around others; hides or discards food

- Purging: uses laxatives, diet pills, ipecac syrup, or water pills; may engage in self-induced vomiting; may run to the bathroom after eating in order to vomit and quickly get rid of the calories (see also bulimia nervosa).
- May engage in frequent, strenuous exercise
- Perception of self to be overweight despite being told by others they are too thin and, in most cases, underweight.
- Becomes intolerant to cold and frequently complains of being cold from loss of insulating body fat or poor circulation resulting from extremely low blood pressure; body temperature lowers (hypothermia) in effort to conserve energy
- Depression: may frequently be in a sad, lethargic state
- Solitude: may avoid friends and family; becomes withdrawn and secretive
- Cheeks may become swollen because of enlargement of the salivary glands caused by excessive vomiting
- Swollen joints
- Abdominal distension
- Bad breath (from vomiting or starvation-induced ketosis)

- Hair loss or thinning
- Fatigue

Some aspects of Anorexia can be experienced during your competition prep, such as the feeling of not being "lean" enough, or feeling too "fat" even though your actual body fat percentage is extremely low. Although your calories do not reflect that of someone going through anorexia, some of the mental and physical aspects of the disorder can become apparent. You might not be "choosing" to live as someone going through anorexia, however the sport of competing can somewhat "force" you to mirror many similar experiences as someone who is dealing with the disease.

The biggest chance of developing this disease is after the competition. Most girls put on a significant amount of weight in a fairly short amount of time post comp, due to resuming a "normal" eating lifestyle. It is absolutely not realistic to maintain the extreme low body fat percentage on a day to day basis, and is completely unrealistic to maintain that expectation once you are no longer following a competition diet. Due to this fact, many girls become "desperate" in their desire to reclaim their competition physique, and thus result to more extreme measures like cutting calories, resuming a comp diet, incorporating extreme amounts of exercise, or a combination of all three. If you find yourself becoming afraid to eat or recognize any of the above signs, please seek the appropriate help. (For the full article, visit

http://en.wikipedia.org/wiki/Anorexia_nervosa)

Bulimia:

Wikipedia defines Bulimia as: Bulimia nervosa is an eating disorder characterized by binge eating and purging, or consuming a large amount of food in a short amount of time followed by an attempt to rid oneself of the food consumed (purging), typically by vomiting, taking a laxative or diuretic, and/or excessive exercise. These acts are also commonly accompanied with fasting over an extended period of time. Bulimia nervosa is considered to be less life threatening than anorexia; however, the occurrence of bulimia nervosa is higher. Bulimia nervosa is nine times more likely to occur in women than men (Barker 2003). The vast majority of those with bulimia nervosa are at normal weight. Antidepressants, especially SSRIs, are widely used in the treatment of bulimia nervosa (Newell and Gournay 2000). Patients who have bulimia nervosa are often linked with having impulsive behaviors involving overspending and sexual behaviors as well as having family histories of alcohol and substance abuse, mood and eating disorders.

These are some of the many signs that may indicate whether someone has bulimia nervosa:

- fixation on amount of calories consumed
- fixated and extremely conscious of weight
- low self-esteem
- low blood pressure
- irregular menstrual cycle
- constant trips to the bathroom
- depression

Bulimia and binge eating can become prevalent in competition prep (or afterwards) in order to achieve the feeling of being "full" without any calorie repercussions. I've come across many girls during their extreme dieting, resort to a little bite of something "forbidden" only to find their self totally immersed in a full blown binge. Although not all girls choose to purge (or throw up) afterwards, some will try to compensate by skipping meals or by participating in excessive exercising.

I believe that binge eating can become very dominant during competition prep, even among girls who have never experienced this disorder prior to competing. Most often some of the subtle signs of binge eating become apparent once a competitor is allowed a "cheat meal" and able to eat whatever they want (and how much they want) for that specific meal. Personally, I found a direct correlation between how deprived/hungry I felt to how much food was consumed during a scheduled cheat. It became common for me to indulge in extremely large amounts of food, pushing my body to the point of feeling nauseated and over stuffed. Although this is "allowed" during a cheat, be diligent in making sure this action does not carry on into your daily routine. As with any disorder, if you feel you are experiencing any signs or symptoms of Bulimia or Binge Eating please contact a professional. (The full article can be read at

http://en.wikipedia.org/wiki/Bulimia)

Depression:

We all go through ups and downs in our mood. Sadness is a normal reaction to life's struggles, setbacks, and disappointments. Many people use the word "depression" to explain these kinds of feelings, but depression is much more than just sadness. Coming off of the "high" of competing, especially when it has consumed a good amount of your energy, time, and thoughts can easily leave you with an "empty" or "now what?" feeling. I have personally witnessed a handful of women who were not prepared for the letdown after their competition was over, the weight gain associated with off season, or the lack of structure slip into depression.

Wikipedia describes depression as: Depression is a state of low mood and aversion to activity that can have a negative effect on a person's thoughts, behavior, feelings, world view and physical well-being. Depressed people may feel sad, anxious, empty, hopeless, worried, helpless, worthless, guilty, irritable, hurt, or restless. They may lose interest in activities that once were pleasurable; experience loss of appetite or overeating; have problems concentrating, remembering details, or making decisions; and may contemplate or attempt suicide. Insomnia, excessive sleeping, fatigue, loss of energy, or aches, pains or digestive problems that are resistant to treatment may be present. (The full article can be found at http://en.wikipedia.org/wiki/Depression_(mood))

The best way to avoid experiencing depression after your show is to be prepared for the "off season." An excellent way to achieve this is to set goals you would like to achieve during the time you are not competing. It can also be extremely beneficial to have an eating plan in order so you will feel some sense of structure once you enter the off season. Although it is normal to experience somewhat of emptiness or loss of direction after your competition season has come to an end, it is important to seek help if you feel yourself becoming increasingly depressed.

Body Dysmorphic Disorder:

Although many of the above topics are more of a reaction to Body Dysmorphic Disorder (BDD), I wanted to talk about this disorder on its own as I believe this is the disorder with the highest probability of being experienced by a competitor. During prep, competitors take their body fat levels to very low percentages, usually lower than what they have ever experienced. Over time, seeing the muscles emerge, the abs become visible, and your whole body morph into this extreme state, it can be very easy to forget what "normal" looks like. You become accustomed to your "new" body and thus start raising the bar on your expectations for what you should look like on a day to day basis.

Wikipedia defines some characteristics of BDD as follows: BDD is often misunderstood as a vanity-driven obsession, whereas it is quite the opposite; people with BDD do not believe themselves to be better looking than others, but instead feel that their perceived "defect" is irrevocably ugly or not good enough. People with BDD may compulsively look at themselves in the mirror or, conversely, cover up and avoid mirrors. They typically think about their appearance for at least one hour a day (and usually more) and, in severe cases, may drop all social contact and responsibilities as they become a recluse.

Common symptoms of BDD include:

- Obsessive thoughts about (a) perceived appearance defect(s).
- Obsessive and compulsive behaviors related to (a) perceived appearance defect(s) (see section below).
- Major depressive disorder symptoms.
- Delusional thoughts and beliefs related to (a) perceived appearance defect(s).
- Social and family withdrawal, social phobia, loneliness and self-imposed social isolation.
- Suicidal ideation.
- Anxiety; possible panic attacks.
- Chronic low self-esteem.
- Feeling self-conscious in social environments; thinking that others notice and mock their perceived defect(s).
- Strong feelings of shame.

- Avoidant personality: avoiding leaving the home or only leaving the home at certain times.
- Dependent personality: dependence on others, such as a partner, friend or family.
- Inability to work or an inability to focus at work due to preoccupation with appearance.
- Problems initiating and maintaining relationships (both intimate relationships and friendships).
- Alcohol and/or drug abuse (often an attempt to self-medicate).
- Repetitive behavior (such as constantly (and heavily) applying make-up; regularly checking appearance in mirrors; see section below for more associated behavior).
- Seeing slightly varying image of self upon each instance of observing a mirror or reflective surface.
- Perfectionism (undergoing cosmetic surgery and behaviors such as excessive moisturizing and exercising with the aim to achieve an ideal body type and reduce anxiety).

Note: any kind of body modification may change one's appearance. There are many types of body modification that do not include surgery/cosmetic surgery. Body modification (or related behavior) may seem compulsive, repetitive, or focused on one or more areas or features that the individual perceives to be defective.

Common compulsive behaviors associated with BDD include:

- Compulsive mirror checking, glancing in reflective doors, windows and other reflective surfaces.
- Alternatively, inability to look at one's own reflection or photographs of oneself; also, removal of mirrors from the home.
- Attempting to camouflage the imagined defect: for example, using cosmetic camouflage, wearing baggy clothing, maintaining specific body posture or wearing hats.
- Use of distraction techniques to divert attention away from the person's perceived defect, e.g. wearing extravagant clothing or excessive jewelry.
- Excessive grooming behaviors: skin-picking, combing hair, plucking eyebrows, shaving, etc.
- Compulsive skin-touching, especially to measure or feel the perceived defect.
- Unmotivated hostility toward people, especially those of the opposite sex (or same sex if

homosexual).

- Seeking reassurance from loved ones.
- Excessive dieting or exercising, working on outside appearance.
- Self-harm.
- Comparing appearance/body parts with that/those of others, or obsessive viewing of favorite celebrities or models whom the person suffering from BDD wishes to resemble.
- Compulsive information-seeking: reading books, newspaper articles and websites that relate to the person's perceived defect, e.g. losing hair or being overweight.
- Obsession with plastic surgery or dermatological procedures, often with little satisfactory results (in the perception of the patient). In extreme cases, patients have attempted to perform plastic surgery on themselves, including liposuction and various implants, with disastrous results.
- Excessive enema use (if obesity is the concern).

(To access the full article, visit http://en.wikipedia.org/wiki/Body_dismorphic_disorder)

I cannot stress this enough: YOUR COMPETITION PHYSIQUE IS **TEMPORARY!** It is not a realistic expectation to walk around year round with an extremely low body fat percentage and can be harmful to your body's natural hormonal state. If you can come to terms with the fact that gaining weight post comp is a natural part of the competition cycle, you will have an easier time accepting the changes to your physique. Again, proper planning BEFORE you enter your off season can better equip you in dealing with post comp body issues. As with everything else, if you feel you are struggling with BDD, contact a professional.

Final Note:

I believe it is very important to discuss eating issues and body image disorders when it comes to competing. Although no one wants to believe they will experience any negative effect from competing, I would be neglectful in equipping you with every aspect of the competition process if I did not at least present the topic as a possibility. Getting ready for a show can be a great experience, and is, for many. If you are aware of possibilities that could arise during and post comp, you can at least prepare and educate yourself in order to ward off any negative feelings or emotions that could arise. Again, reminding yourself that competing puts your body into various cycles and phases (not just lean all the time) and is all part of the whole process, you can enjoy every phase and feel confident in your changing body.

Chapter 15

Final Words

I hope this book has provided you with a wealth of information, resources and tips regarding the ins and outs of competing. As I stated in the beginning of the book, I truly believe this book has been a project seven years in the making. Over the years I have learned many little tricks or tidbits of information that have helped me improve everything from my physique to my stage presence, which has made for a very memorable and successful competing experience.

Although I have done my best to address every aspect of competing I could think of, I do realize there are certain elements to this sport that can be learned only through EXPERIENCING the whole process. I cannot tell you which trainer or diet best suits you, I cannot suggest the best color of suit to wear, nor can I write about which of the talked about experiences you will actually encounter. My goal was not to be your personal trainer, yet merely to prepare you with knowledge regarding certain aspects of competing.

This book was written for YOU, out of my desire to provide a comprehensive resource for any female competitor to have access to. It was my love of the sport, combined with my love of helping others become successful in as short amount of time as possible that gave birth to this book. I remember, seven years ago, looking for a book or guide to help me answer all the questions/topics covered in this book, yet could not find all of this information in one spot. During those years, I spent many hours scouring the web for the best resources, and went through numerous competitions to learn anything and everything I could that would help me in this sport. After interacting with many female competitors over the years I realized that, like me, there are numerous girls out there who wish they could get a compilation of information, without bias, in one basic spot.

Over the years I have also been very blessed with meeting some amazing competitors and judges. I truly believe that though other people's accounts in this chosen sport, we can further our knowledge and camaraderie by sharing our stories, mistakes, tips, and overall experiences. I wish I had known a competitor and/or judge when I was starting out that could say, "Ok, this is what you need to know," or, "This is what I went through, just so you know."

It is because of my belief that knowledge is a key component in being successful, and the desire of some amazing competitors and judges to ensure you are well quipped and prepared for this sport, that I am able to provide Q and A sections with: Judges, Competitors, a Professional Photographer, and Competitors dealing with eating/body image disorders. (Some names have been changed to protect identity) They have each taken the time to answer my questions as openly, honestly, and thoroughly as they can in order to provide you with a wealth of information. I hope you can get further insight into the world of competing through their eyes.

In closing, I would like to personally thank you for purchasing this book and sincerely hope you have received an enormous wealth of information. I am passionate about providing the most unbiased, current, and important details to you, in hopes of being even a small part of your success in this sport. Best of luck to you on your journey, no matter which part of it you are on. May you always make, "First Call Out."

Chapter 16

Q & A

Part 1: Disorders

What disorder(s) do you currently/or have in the past dealt with? (Anorexia, Binge Eating, Body Image Disorder)

Anorexia (when I was a young teen, before I discovered the "magic" of bulimia.)

Bulimia: have struggled with this disorder throughout my whole life. I was anorexic/bulimic as a teenager and throughout my early twenties.

Binge Eating: food is my DRUG. I use food as a way to comfort, to cope. When the guilt of a binge settles in, I turn to the practice of my bulimia and purge. Other times, I will punish myself, and allow the guilt to contain me while NOT purging; perhaps to remind myself why binging is bad. There's always the "I will NEVER do this ever again" factor that I feel after a binge. I usually binge in secret.

Body Image Disorder: Yep, I have it. I am certain that almost every woman that has one of the listed disorders has warped ideas of what their bodies look like. I am currently struggling with the off-season look that I am currently sporting. I try not to use negative self-talk these days, but it's hard not to feel "fat" and "gross" when I can no longer wear the skinny, pre-competition clothes that my closet is full of.

How long have you had this disorder?

I have struggled with my weight my whole life! It has constantly yo-yoed. However, my eating disordered life was born at the brink of my high-school career. I didn't want to be a fat freshman!

Let's talk about competing and how your disorder kind of played into the whole process. If you had the disorder prior to entering your first competition, did you consider what role the disorder would play during your prep?

I honestly believed that the whole competition process would actually help keep my disordered eating at bay. A meal plan, professional coaching staff to keep my accountable, living constantly in the gym: these are all things that I thought would hinder any binging, purging, or anorexic behavior. I almost felt a sense of relief with the meal plan: I had an exact plan! I wouldn't have to worry about choosing the "wrong" type of food!

If you worked with a trainer, were they aware of your struggles?

When I had my initial interview with the team of coaches that trained me for me first couple of shows, I was very sure that they were aware that I used to have a weight issue, and that eating disorders were such a huge part of my life. Oddly enough, up until I began training for my first figure competition, I hadn't "relapsed" with my eating disorders for the better part of a year. It wasn't until I was in my second month of training that food began to look both forbidden and magical.

If yes, what did you say to them and what was their response?

Come to think of it, there wasn't much OF a response. I remember a coach saying, "well....it looks like you don't have an issue with food anymore", which at the time, I took as both an insult and a relief that it wasn't going to be discussed anymore. Talk to these "strangers" about my food issues? I would rather have teeth pulled!

If no, why didn't you address the topic?

N/A

Speaking personally, having suffered with anorexia and body image disorder for about 20 years now, I kind of used competition prep as a more "acceptable" outlet for my disorders. Do you think

your decision to compete had anything to do with trying to find an "outlet" so to speak? If so, how?

Yes. At the time, I hadn't really given it much thought, because, as it was my first go-around with competing, I honestly had NO idea how much the diet played into the final show-ready physique. I remember telling my husband during the first month of rigid show prep that I felt that this program would "keep me on my toes", and my "hand out of the cookie jar". I had forgotten what extreme hunger felt like up until that point. I thought that I had found a temporary "cure" for my binge eating disorder. I felt, rather, that I had WON, beating my eating disorders, leaving in them in the past as I started my show prep...it wasn't until much later into my training that I realized how dead wrong I was.

Did you have any struggles during your prep due to disorder? Any relapses?

I first began to get somewhat lax with my diet the second month into training. The new diet actually had me GAINING weight, and while I knew that some of it could be muscle, and though I knew that I was eating more quality food than I was previously to contest prep, I felt DEPRESSED. I began to drop weight again, and with that, I felt that I may have some "freedom" with the diet. I ate an extra serving of "legal" carbs or protein here and there, or when I made my husband his lunch for work, I may have more than occasionally helped myself to a potato chip (or two, or three, or seven!).

My husband and I are very social people, and when I began having to answer no to invites from friends that were having parties, barbeques, I became more and more resentful at the diet and at myself for having decided to put myself and my husband through what seemed like a ridiculous diet. I remember hearing my husband mention to other people how strict that my diet was, that "My wife is getting only enough food just to survive". A bit extreme, but it felt rather legit.

If bulimic answer: Did you have any relapses or episodes during your prep? Would you be willing to share a "typical" occurrence?

If anorexic answer: I tell people that anorexia is actually easier because after not eating for so long, the hunger signal actually goes away. However, when comp dieting and eating every three hours your hunger is constantly being fueled. Due to this, when I DID get a cheat meal, I started binge eating for fear of starvation. Did you experience anything similar? Anything you can add?

I had small relapses here and there throughout the

majority of my contest prep. However, the MAJOR relapses left me feeling drained, dead, ready to quit. I knew that I was heading into disaster when ALL THAT I COULD THINK ABOUT WAS FOOD. Nothing was more important than what I would/could eat after my show. Every Wednesday, my mailbox would be full of the grocery store's food mailers for the week...I would sit, leaf through every single one of them, pathetically staring and drooling over pictures of food. The people in the ads always looked so happy, a smile on their faces as they indulged in a grilled hamburger at the backyard BBQ. Jealous? Yes. It fueled a certain anger/jealousy combo that I hadn't felt since I was child, when my grandmother told me that I couldn't have any chocolate because I was fat.

The major binge eating experience that comes to mind was right before my second show. I was at the gym; it was the dreaded leg day. I pushed my weak, carb-depleted body too hard, and fainted in the ladies locker room. A woman gave me a granola bar, was given some juice, and I remember feeling more AMAZING at the sugar flowing through my veins than guilty for "cheating" on my diet. I left the gym wanting MORE. I stopped at the gas station, got a diet orange soda, king-sized packages of peanut M&M's and Reese's

Peanut Butter Cups. I went back to my car, opened the packages with mad fury, and remember just completely numbing out as I savored every bite of my own personal chocolate heaven. I experienced a sugar buzz, was on cloud nine....it was a feeling of euphoria, and I couldn't stop. I figured, "you've already cheated this terribly on your diet, why stop now?"....I put my car into drive, and headed to Wendy's for a huge double cheeseburger, large fried, and a sugar-filled Coca Cola. I downed that meal so quickly, that I doubt if I even tasted it. The grand finale was another drive, this time to Sheridan's for a large concrete LOADED with candy. After I inhaled that, the guilt and the physical pain of my now-distended belly kicked in. I ate so much, that it hurt to even DRIVE.

As soon as I got back to my house, I made a beeline directly for the bathroom, and I purged. Hands down: the worst binging and purging episode of my life happened that day.

When it was all over, I sobbed.

For all:

Do you feel like competition prep intensified your problems? If so, how?

Most definitely. Competing places a magnifying glass over eating disorders, and brings the little sleeping devils out to play, no matter HOW long they may or may not have remained dormant. This is a very serious issue that I fully believe needs to be discussed with every woman before she ever gets ready to begin a competition career.

Did you develop any new disorder (like body image disorder) as a result of competing? Can you discuss?

I believe that prior to competing, that I was disordered on views with how I perceived my body to look. However, since competing, my self-views on my appearance are night and day. While some days are better than others (there are moments where I just want to be shed of this muscle and be "little and skinny" again), I struggle the most with how I feel in my new off-season skin. I use negative self-talk far too often, especially when I attempt to squeeze into a pair of pants that I used to wear before competition training and they don't fit. A size 0 to a 4/6 isn't terrible, but feels like a huge shift in size when you have terrible body image issues. I need to look at it as a reason to go shopping, to find clothes that fit my more muscular, fit bod, rather than beat myself up for not fitting into a waif's skinny jeans!

Many girls don't realize what is going to happen

once the competition is over and there is no "structure" to their nutrition plan. The effect that has on your body can be quite the shock, especially for those who deal with body image issues. Can you share what your post comp experience was and how you coped?

I will admit that walking around lean and sporting a six-pack sure did make the competition worth it at times. However, it is unhealthy and unrealistic to try to maintain that level of leanness year-round. When my final show was over, I remember the relief of having survived, that I could now "live a little". This is where my old ways of binging caught up with me to a level of madness: I began eating EVERYTHING in sight. In a way, it was almost like I was eating out of sheer anger... "You told me that I couldn't eat this, well...watch me eat it now!" I ate food that I never really even typically liked, just to taste it. I went to a countless number of buffets just to experience the ecstasy that usually comes along with gluttony; cakes, brownies, pizza, cheeseburgers, loaded baked potatoes...you name it, I at least had several bites just to "taste it". It was almost like I had been locked inside of a starvation camp for months, and now that I was seeing the light of day, I went absolutely mad. I gained

30 pounds in a matter of a month. Even my poor husband put on sympathy weight, and is still working to lose those extra pounds that he put on post-show. Not going into an off-season geared with the right tools is a set up for disaster, but it is ultimately up to the competitor on whether or not she applies the off-season dietary tools into her diet. I, myself, had the knowledge on how to eat, however: I wasn't ready. I perhaps needed to gain that weight, to see the weight gain, to feel like crap, before I was ready to hop back on the diet bandwagon.

Any final thoughts, comments, or pieces of advice you would be willing to share?

To never be afraid to reach out to another person and discuss how you're feeling and your behaviors towards food while undergoing a tough-as-nails competition training program. Support from others will keep you sane.

Knowing that I wasn't alone, that I wasn't some kind of "freak" or a failure gave me hope to keep going forward and to prove to myself that I was a true champion at heart: food wasn't going to defeat me!

Thank you!!

What disorder(s) do you currently/or have in the past dealt with? (Anorexia, Binge Eating, Body Image Disorder)

Body Image Disorder

How long have you had this disorder?

Pretty much all my life…I have always carried quite a bit of muscle for a girl, athletic build. As a young girl and a teenager, I hated it! I remember all through high school, wearing shirts that were long enough to cover my biceps, because I was ashamed of looking like a boy and hated that when I looked down I could see the muscles on the sides of my legs. But in the two years it has gotten worse, since the dieting, tracking fat %, weight and etc…all that goes along with competing. Although as I've gotten older I have learned to appreciate all the things I hated as I was growing up. I've learned that muscle is a good thing to have, and a lot of women cannot get it, hard as they try. I now love my arms, and my legs. But like I said now, I just want it to be more…and I don't know why.

Let's talk about competing and how your disorder kind of played into the whole process. If you had the disorder prior to entering your first competition, did you consider what role the disorder would play during your prep?

I've never really like hated my body, have always been athletic, and have actually liked the way my body is…but always feel that it can be improved. Since the competitions with my body fat percentage being so low for so long, I always feel now like what used to be normal is not good enough anymore. I want my body fat numbers to be one digit, like they were before…even though I'm not competing. Even being at 12% and 135 lbs. where I am now, I feel fat, and feel like I'm not good enough.

If you worked with a trainer, were they aware of your struggles?

I only had a trainer for one day a week for two months, and he is more or less just my friend, so he just tells me flat out, "You need to eat more…take care of yourself; you're too skinny." (He doesn't like me that way!) You need to eat more…take care of yourself, he tells me. He has always told me I need to see what other people see, that I am beautiful and he can't believe that I can't see that. He is one that first mentioned the thought of me competing in figure, and since my first show, he has absolutely hated it! He doesn't want me to compete; he hates what it does to my body. He thinks I look best where I am right now. I just have to try to believe him and trust him, hard as it is for me. I don't like where I am now!

If yes, what did you say to them and what was their response?

N/A

If no, why didn't you address the topic? I never realized I had a problem until the last year.

N/A

Speaking personally, having suffered with anorexia and body image disorder for about 20 years now, I kind of used competition prep as a more "acceptable" outlet for my disorders. Do you think your decision to compete had anything to do with trying to find an "outlet" so to speak? If so, how?

No, I only did the competition; because the trainer and another friend had mentioned it several times to me that my body was made for it, great muscle tone etc. I only did it to say that I did and to conquer my fear of being on stage in front of hundreds of people, because I have always been shy, and very self-conscious. I have been that way my whole life. I think it stems from having a family that thinks it's funny to laugh and ridicule, (my dad and my brother) saying I'm fat, when I'm not. Even when I was 115 lbs, and 6% body fat, my Dad saw a pic of me on my computer and laughed and said, "Look how wide you are in that picture, God Sis!" That hurts me so bad, because I have always been the only athletic one in my family and I work hard. They never told me I was too skinny, so I still felt like I was not good enough. I wanted to be more, and still want to be leaner.

Did you have any struggles during your prep due to disorder? Any relapses?

My prep was much easier I think than other women that have done these competitions. I don't know if it has to do with great metabolism or what, but I never had to do a lot of cardio, always had my cheat at least once a week, and kept my apple and peanut butter all the way up to week before.

If bulimic answer: Did you have any relapses or episodes during your prep? Would you be willing to share a "typical" occurrence?

N/A

If anorexic answer: I tell people that anorexia is actually easier because after not eating for so long, the hunger signal actually goes away. However, when comp dieting and eating every three hours your hunger is constantly being fueled. Due to this, when I DID get a cheat meal, I started binge eating for fear of starvation. Did you experience

anything similar? Anything you can add?

For all: I have never been anorexic or bulimic. But after competing and being on pretty strict diet for a year and a half, I binged on food immediately after my show. After one of my shows, (when I was 6% body fat and 113 lbs) I went to Sonic and had a large Oreo Blast, a Supersonic Bacon Cheeseburger, large fries, and a large drink. I ate all of it, then two hours later I had food delivered to my room, which included: chicken strips, fries, salad with lots of Ranch dressing, large piece of carrot cake, red velvet cake, several candy bars, more pop and tons of water. Again this was within a few hours before going to bed that night. I felt like I couldn't get enough to eat and that I was starving. Within 3 days I had gained 20 lbs.

Do you feel like competition prep intensified your problems? If so, how?

Yes! I had never been a bad eater, always pretty healthy, and hardly any candy and such. If I had stuck to more of the way I've always eaten instead of changing things so drastically from July-Oct. I don't think my weight or body fat would have dropped so dangerously low, and my eating would be under control now. Things that I never wanted before comp, I now crave all the time, such as chocolate and ice cream.

Did you develop any new disorder (like body image disorder) as a result of competing? Can you discuss?

Yes, again after looking a certain way for competition it is so hard to go back to the way you used to be, which is normal. I wanted to feel like I did before (being lean), but with the extra body fat and weight, plus not competing, I felt fat, disgusting and just not good enough!

Many girls don't realize what is going to happen once the competition is over and there is no "structure" to their nutrition plan. The effect that has on your body can be quite the shock, especially for those who deal with body image issues. Can you share what your post comp experience was and how you coped?

It is so hard to go from seeing a lean, little body (stage) to a normal, everyday body that you will have after. It has been a year since I competed and I still struggle daily, looking in the mirror and trying to accept that this is how I'm supposed to look. My husband tells me I have "anorexic eyes" and that I can't see who I am. He tells me I am beautiful, and was just too skinny during competition. I'm eating whatever I want, and although I love the food, there are days where I try to make up for the day before by eating only salads, and exercising more. I still take a thermogenic once a day and have never stopped taking them in a year and a half. My multivitamin has a metabolism booster in it; I take water pills often, drink coffee, green tea, and grapefruit juice. Even though I'm not competing, I also still consume my protein and BCAA'S every day.

Any final thoughts, comments, or pieces of advice you would be willing to share?

My only reason for ever going to the gym after not using the gym membership for 3 years was to be healthy again; I just wanted to tone up. My dream weight was to be 125 lbs. again. I had been through a lot of death in my family as well as friends in 2 short years. I didn't realize that going through depression affected the immune system until I kept getting recurring infections. At one point while whitewater rafting in Colorado, I became extremely sick with diarrhea to the point that I had to quit my job. It went on for 2 ½ years. After seeing several doctors, having tons of tests performed repeatedly and numerous antibiotics for infections, the internal doctor finally diagnosed it with Giardia (parasites) from the waters in Colorado. The reason I had it and no one else did was due to my immune system shutting down from dealing with all the stress in my life. Long story I know, but I joined the gym to relieve stress, just to feel good again; never in a million years did I ever imagine or dream I would be a Figure competitor. Although I had never even heard of Figure before, I am so glad I did it. My first one will always be one of my proudest moments. The pride you feel for yourself, the hard work, the dedication, the sacrifices that you make to get to be on that stage… I would not trade it for anything in the world. I met so many wonderful people, who I still talk to all the time and I will always cherish that. But, I do feel like competing can be taken to extremes as in the case of my second competition.

Although it was only 2 months after my first one, it was one I really didn't want to do, but was basically talked into it. I was already at 9-10% body fat, 120 lbs. but started a drastic a new diet to get to where I thought I needed to be due to being told I was not lean enough. After all of the dieting I only got 5[th,] but I kept going and going until I was at 113 lbs., and 6% body fat. Through the whole process I couldn't see what I really was in the mirror anymore. Even though I took progress pictures weekly, and still to this day to see where I am at, I still want more, and feel like I'm never good enough! I'm still struggling to be comfortable with what used to be my ideal body. I look better than I ever have, so people say, (just not stage ready) but I still can't see what other people see and no matter how hard I try I can't be completely happy with what I see. You can use anything I send you or nothing at all, but this is something that I wrote awhile back.

Only in competition do we choose to be judged on our bodies, but outside in real life also, we are constantly judged as being too heavy, too thin, best legs, best butt, prettiest face, prettiest smile, fit or not fit. We all have issues with our self-image and have to deal with it. Just because you see or think one way, does not mean that everyone else agrees. Humans by nature judge others…that's just what we do, and it's not right. It is often jealousy and insecurities that spark criticism and negativity. We should all celebrate and appreciate our differences (our own bodies) as we strive to be healthy and fit, and aim for happiness. I saw this on a friend's page a long time ago and I love it: My definition of competition?

Always living with a feeling of doubt and inferiority? True winners don't compete, they evolve. Stop competing and comparing. Keep evolving and become your own beautiful creation!

Thank You!

What disorder(s) do you currently/or have in the past dealt with? (Anorexia, Binge Eating, Body Image Disorder)

Anorexia Nervosa /purging type as well

How long have you had this disorder?

Since 2006.

Let's talk about competing and how your disorder kind of played into the whole process. If you had the disorder prior to entering your first competition, did you consider what role the disorder would play during your prep?

I did my first competition 9 months after my daughter was born. I had such a hard time during pregnancy dealing with my body changing and gaining weight that my initial instinct was to go right back into my eating disorder. I have always worked out daily and had known girls who had turned their lives around getting into competing once they had overcome their eating disorders. My trainer that I had worked with throughout my pregnancy thought it would be a good idea to actually help me realize that I HAD to eat in order to get the body I desired. My therapist thought it might be good for me as well to help me lose my baby weight in a more healthy fashion, or so we thought.

If you worked with a trainer, were they aware of your struggles? I did let my trainer know about my past history with my eating disorder. He had actually been the head trainer in the gym that I had always gone to and had seen me at my lowest weight. He promised to work with me following my show to help me get back to a normal life. Unfortunately, that in turn is not what happened either time. I was left on my own and my eating disorder spun out of control.

If yes, what did you say to them and what was their response?

I just told them the condition of me doing a show was that they work with me when it had completed and that I needed a maintenance diet. I did not want to be weighed every day or have my body fat tested.

If no, why didn't you address the topic?

Speaking personally, having suffered with anorexia and body image disorder for about 20 years now, I kind of used competition prep as a more "acceptable" outlet for my disorders. Do you think your decision to compete had anything to do with trying to find an "outlet" so to speak? If so, how?

It definitely did. It allowed me to have a "reason" to diet and only eat what was acceptable on my comp diet. It also allowed me to get very thin without everyone wanting to put me back in treatment. It was really a way to fool my family into thinking I was ok when I knew I really wasn't.

Did you have any struggles during your prep due to disorder? Any relapses?

I purged several times during my comp prep. It typically was when I was extremely hungry and would allow myself a couple of extra bites or ounces of something. I had to find a way to get "rid of it" so purging made me feel like I could get the control back. I felt like I was weak because I couldn't follow the competition diet exactly as I should when other girls out there probably did it flawlessly. I would also not eat my meals at the times I should because I thought I can stand this hungry feeling until later in the morning because it allows me to "conserve more food" for later.

If bulimic answer: Did you have any relapses or episodes during your prep? Would you be willing to share a "typical" occurrence?

If anorexic answer:

I tell people that anorexia is actually easier because after not eating for so long, the hunger signal actually goes away. However, when comp

dieting and eating every three hours your hunger is constantly being fueled. Due to this, when I DID get a cheat meal, I started binge eating for fear of starvation. Did you experience anything similar? Anything you can add?

I was never allowed any cheat meals but I definitely agree that the hunger signals due to eating every three hours were something I had never experienced and it caused me anxiety. So much so that I was medicated and now have severe anxiety disorder that I will need medication for probably forever.

For all:

Do you feel like competition prep intensified your problems? If so, how?

It definitely intensified my issues. I wanted that stage body every day. That water depleted, tiny body every day of my life. I know in my mind you can't live in that body but I was willing to try. After both of my shows I would go through the week living on just enough food to get by and fat burners and the weekends I would binge and purge out of control. I feel like I have lost all perception of what health really is. You look at the girls training for these shows, working out endless hours and being so disciplined in their eating and you think they are the portrait of health when in all honesty they are just another person living a disorder.

Did you develop any new disorder (like body image disorder) as a result of competing? Can you discuss?

Body image disorder was always a part of my anorexia but I can definitely say it intensified to new levels after competing. I began to see "fat" in places I never would have really thought about on my worst day in my anorexic body. I had just added a fuel to the fire I definitely did not need to add.

Many girls don't realize what is going to happen once the competition is over and there is no "structure" to their nutrition plan. The effect that has on your body can be quite the shock, especially for those who deal with body image issues. Can you share what your post comp experience was and how you coped?

I went to therapy biweekly throughout both of my competition preps as I have done for the past 5 years. We discussed prior to the show what the plan was for me and how I would handle coming down from the high of the show. Both times I failed. I ended up binging and purging, restricting, and spending ridiculous amounts of time in the gym. After you do a show you think people look at you every time they see you like "wow she got fat after her show" I feel additional pressure since my trainer is at my gym every single day. I felt like I was a failure like I had let him down not being able to maintain the body I had worked so hard to achieve. Anti- depressants were prescribed both times and help take the edge of but nothing makes the thoughts go away.

Any final thoughts, comments, or pieces of advice you would be willing to share?

In my honest opinion fitness shows are just an arena for disordered people. I know they say "if it was easy everyone would do it" but in all honesty that isn't it at all. The experience in doing a show is great. The girls are great but at what cost? I have known plenty of friends who have never had an eating disorder who have come to me in private following a show to ask me for advice. I think the best advice I have is to stay away. Don't do it. You can have a fit healthy body without going to these extremes and draining yourself both physically and emotionally. In the end it just isn't worth it.

Thank you!!

Chapter 17

Q &A

Part 2: Competitors

Name: Jennifer Isenberg

Division you compete in: Women's Physique and masters women's physique

Organization(s) you compete in: NPC

Number of years competed: less than 1

Competition weight: 132#

Off season weight: 155#

What made you decide to compete?

I'm going to start this off with a little history on me—I began to work out about 5 years ago, only when I wasn't hung over or out partying. I have been drinking/partying since I was 15, and became sober 1 year ago September 2011. I have gotten into every kind of physical contest and challenge since from mud runs, biking, rock climbing, yoga to half marathons. But I really enjoy lifting heavy, and bodybuilding has become a huge part of my sober life! My boyfriend introduced me to shows and competitions, after watching him on stage a few times; I got bit by the show bug!

I chose physique, because my body type is an easy gainer of muscle and I really like lifting heavy with my man. It just fit how I like to work out. I also picked physique over figure because I liked the idea of posing and the routine! Felt like I could bring my personality on stage with me!

In preparation for your first show, how long did you train for? If you have competed since, has the time required to prep changed at all? If so, how?

I have only done one show so far…I dieted for 15 weeks. Looking back on it now, I also realized that I have only been working out/lifting seriously meaning drug and alcohol free for 7months prior to when I began dieting. I have always been on a fat burning diet of some sort, and have never been on a muscle building diet/plan. I kind of jumped in to doing a show with not enough background. I am planning to do a show one year from my first. This time I'm giving my body plenty of rebuild/repair time and more time to drop my body fat.

How did you choose a trainer?

My boyfriend competes and I used his friend/trainer Kit

Kittson from In shape Nutrition. He is awesome! Very knowledgeable, patient seems like he truly cares about the mental and the physical aspects!

What do you think is an important, or the most important, thing to consider when trying to find a trainer?

Reputation, honesty on whether or not your ideas will translate to the stage. And that your trainers program is realistic—amount of cardio/time in the gym to diet being not too extreme. That they train the entire package-mind and body.

I mention in the book that I consider this sport to be kind of a 'selfish' sport. I've given my point of view on this subject. Do you agree? If so, can you explain how leading a competition prep life interferes with "normal" life? How did you cope with that? What is best piece of advice you can give to competitors regarding this aspect?

I got to experience this on both sides! My boyfriend has done 3 competitions prior to the one we did together.

When he was prepping… he was crabby, distant and I couldn't wait till we got back to "us" because it was so focused on him…what he could eat, where he could go, when and how he could work out. By his third show this wasn't so extreme…so it got better.

For my first show, we did it together. Granted he had very little dieting to do, but this way our workouts, diet, cheat meals, and prep mirrored each other. However this made for a messy house, since neither of us had the energy to be much of a housekeeper!

Since we were very self- focused…neither of us felt like we were ignored or lacked attention from the other! We also have a few friends that compete, so spending time with them for socialization made situations easier.

What was hard was family parties, work parties etc…it was difficult to watch everyone else eat all the food while I sat and ate my chicken and veggies. However with that being said, I always planned a meal during those times so that I had something to eat.

The other hard part was not being able to do other activities with my friends like mountain biking, running, spinning, rock climbing. It made me question whether or not this was worth it!

Having a supportive partner is crucial to this, or being single would work! I do believe that through this process you need to show your loved ones appreciation for their support…even if it means writing yourself a reminder to do something nice! Also remember it is easier to walk away then say something you may regret later! I found we both could be irritable and had a pact if one of us walks away, let them go and cool off...even if it's over nothing!

I've also stated that this sport is not cheap! Would you please give an estimate of cost for each of the following:

Super expensive! I also cut back some of the hours I worked which hurt the pocket book even more!

Trainer: $50/week for 15 weeks= $750

Weekly grocery bill: $80- this isn't much different than normal grocery bill though

Posing: $100 for routine

Tanning: $100 only do spray tan for the competition—I had skin cancer and do not tan

Nails: $ 50

Hair: $80

Makeup: $100

Suit: $500

Shoes: None

Entry fees (include organizational membership

fees): $200

Anything I missed: Black outfit to wear after I spray tanned = $80

Supplements: $460

Hotel: $150

After show chow fest: $80

Jewelry: $60

Transportation to show: $80

What surprised you the most going through your first preparation?

How mentally forgetful and slow I became from carb depletion! And how much strength I lost.

What was the most difficult part?

The lifestyle change and the post competition time. Also worrying that I wasn't going to lose enough body fat(self- doubt).

What do you wish you had known prior to comp and during comp prep?

Hmmm…it's hard to say one thing…just going through the process itself seems like I will know more what to expect! I'm a hard core researcher-and I branched out and talked to other competitors to learn, so I feel I went into this pretty prepared!

Let's talk about the dreaded "after the competition." I've seen girls never really recover from the "post comp blues." Did you go through this? How did you cope? Any words of advice to help other girls prepare for the physical/mental changes they will experience "after" the show?

It has been almost two months since my show, and yes I am still in "post comp blues"! After the show, I told myself I could eat whatever I wanted for two days, and then get on a building diet. I ate so much in those two days that I made myself sick! And since haven't been sticking to my diet, even though it has carbs at every meal! I have gained back all of my weight, granted a few pounds is muscle…but it is very hard to look in the mirror now. My self -esteem is low which doesn't help my eating! I do know that some of this is underlying issues from my past that I am working on in counseling! And I know it won't be like this forever! But it is hard! I am really focused on lifting; my strength is ridiculous right now! So much to the point that I am entering a power lifting meet in November!

I think my next show, Instead of going hog wild afterward, I will have a few treats and be done…well that's what I hoping for. My best advice is to have a plan in place for after, and try to mentally prep yourself for the direction of growth and rebuilding afterward!

Just for fun:

What food did you miss most during your competition prep?

Salad and fruit

What was the first thing you ate after the show?

What did I not eat was the better question!! I made oatmeal raisin cookie with caramel apple pie cheesecake filling. My man made us a caramel/toffee/chocolate cheesecake!

What was your favorite competition prep meal?

Oatmeal and veggie omelet…I liked it so much that is was my second meal also! The oatmeal I made with coffee instead of water and added unsweetened Ghirardelli cocoa and Splenda…Delish!

Best part of competing?

Doing my posing and routine on stage! I had a sense of belonging to a group of athletes and enjoyed meeting new people.

Worst part of competing?

Sleeping in your spray tan, not being able to shower before and in between shows, smelling like a farm animal!

Any final advice for potential competitors?

Trust your trainer!! Do not try and do extra cardio or take extra fat burners! Be honest with them…if you relax and just follow the plan, it may help with the stress of it! Don't mix too much caffeine with fat burners! And practice posing early, even though you won't be able to tweak the poses until more muscle definition is there!

Thank you for your time and feedback!!!

Name: Christi Mitchell

Division you compete in: Bodybuilding

Organization(s) you compete in: NANBF & NPC

Number of years competed: 5 years

Competition weight: NANBF 117 NPC 138

Off season weight: 145

What made you decide to compete?

The guy that I worked out with decided to enter his first show, I went and watched and it gave me the itch to try to compete.

In preparation for your first show, how long did you train for?

20 weeks

If you have competed since, has the time required to prep changed at all?

Yes, because I was trying to put on a lot of size, so my off season was a lot of eating and training hard for four months, then the "prep time" was 6 weeks.

If so, how?

How did you choose a trainer?

My "idol" in bodybuilding is Iris Kyle and so I looked her up and ended up having her do my diet and workouts.

What do you think is an important, or the most important, thing to consider when trying to find a trainer?

Being available and being honest and being knowledgeable about the last week of diet.

I mention in the book that I consider this sport to be kind of a 'selfish' sport. I've given my point of view on this subject. Do you agree? If so, can you explain how leading a competition prep life interferes with "normal" life?

Yes! Your social life pretty much comes to an end. You don't have the time nor the energy to go out and do things with people like you normally would. **How did you cope with that?**

I would just have to remind myself that what I am doing is for me and that it's not for the rest of my life, it's just for four or five months out of the year to do something that makes me feel good about myself, and something that I enjoy.

What is best piece of advice you can give to competitors regarding this aspect?

Before you compete, be100% sure that it is what you want to do. Only listen to your trainer's advice and trust in them, because if you don't, you will question everything you are doing.

I've also stated that this sport is not cheap! Would you please give an estimate of cost for each of the following:

Trainer: 3000.00

Weekly grocery bill: 100.00?

Posing: included in the training

Tanning: 50.00

Nails: 50.00

Hair: 120.00

Makeup: 35.00

Suit: 175-300.00

Shoes: 0

Entry fees (include organizational membership fees): 100.00?

Anything I missed:

What surprised you the most going through your first preparation? How different my body would look one day from the next.

What was the most difficult part?

Not being able to eat what I wanted and craved!

What do you wish you had known prior to comp and during comp prep?

How much it was going to cost.

Let's talk about the dreaded "after the competition." I've seen girls never really recover from the "post comp blues." Did you go through this? Yes...

How did you cope?

I had to retrain my mind to think that I couldn't always look competition ready and would take time away from the gym.

Any words of advice to help other girls prepare for the physical/mental changes they will experience "after" the show?

Just remember that your body is going to completely change after your show. It is normal to look "normal" and not so lean all of the time.

Just for fun:

What food did you miss most during your competition prep? Cheeseburgers and Pizza

What was the first thing you ate after the show?

Mexican food

What was your favorite competition prep meal?

Salmon, green Beans and Sweet Potato

Best part of competing?

Looking the best that I have ever looked in my life and knowing that I had the willpower and strength to accomplish one of the most difficult sports around.

Worst part of competing?

Feeling irritable and lethargic

Any final advice for potential competitors?

If you don't think you can do it, buckle down and put all of your effort into it and you will be amazed at what you mind will allow you to do!

Thank you for your time and feedback!!!

Name: Jessica Newman

Division you compete in: Figure

Organization(s) you compete in: NPC & INBF

Number of years competed: 3

Competition weight: 118

Off season weight: 130

What made you decide to compete?

I had a trainer who said you are doing this. So I did it.

In preparation for your first show, how long did you train for? If you have competed since, has the time required to prep changed at all? If so, how?

My first show I trained for 6 weeks. Now its a never ending process and I cut for 8-10 weeks.

How did you choose a trainer?

I watched other girls to see results they got from their trainers.

What do you think is an important, or the most important, thing to consider when trying to find a trainer?

For most of us cost is an issue, this is an expensive sport. Other than that you have to be able to communicate with your trainer.

I mention in the book that I consider this sport to be kind of a 'selfish' sport. I've given my point of view on this subject. Do you agree? If so, can you explain how leading a competition prep life interferes with "normal" life? How did you cope with that? What is best piece of advice you can give to competitors regarding this aspect?

I agree 100%. The dedication it takes to be good at this sport requires you to put training and meals at the top of your priority list. It interferes with almost everything. You can't stay out super late & make early morning workouts. You can't just go order off a menu. Before I start prep for any show I sit down with my kids and we discuss it. We do our best to work around my show schedule for things like vacation.

I've also stated that this sport is not cheap! Would you please give an estimate of cost for each of the following:

Trainer: $1,000.00 /yr

Weekly grocery bill: $150.00

Posing: Included with my training.

Tanning: $85 per show & $30 monthly

Nails: $95 per show

Hair: $55 per show

Makeup: $50

Suit: $1,200.00

Shoes: $45.00

Entry fees (include organizational membership fees):

Depending on number of shows I have spent up to $500.00 a year

Anything I missed:

What surprised you the most going through your first preparation? The dieting. Eating to drop body fat is totally different from eating to lose weight.

What was the most difficult part?

For me it was the isolation I felt first starting out before establishing a network of fellow competitors.

What do you wish you had known prior to comp and during comp prep?

Exactly what to expect. I still wish I had a better grasp on the judging.

Let's talk about the dreaded "after the competition." I've seen girls never really recover from the "post comp blues." Did you go through

this? How did you cope? Any words of advice to help other girls prepare for the physical/mental changes they will experience "after" the show?

That is equal to the worst depression ever. It helps me to choose a new goal and have something to work towards instead of feeling like I'm floating without structure. Keep in mind girls that going from a 24/7 routine to no routine is probably the biggest struggle for all of us. The fact that you work so hard for so long to get that stage body only to have it for a little while seems to send us into shock of some sort.

Just for fun:

What food did you miss most during your competition prep? Breadsticks, you can smell those things for miles.

What was the first thing you ate after the show?

I always stash a bag of candy for after finals.

What was your favorite competition prep meal?

Egg whites, oatmeal and grapefruit.

Best part of competing?

The total control you have over your body

Worst part of competing?

The stress you allow yourself to feel over being judged.

Any final advice for potential competitors?

This isn't something most people do & then walk away from. Once you start you will probably be hooked. Go into it knowing this will be a lifestyle change.

Thank you for your time and feedback!!!

Name: Alyssa Stroud

Division you compete in: Female Bodybuilding

Organization(s) you compete in: NPC

Number of years competed: This was my 6th Year

Competition weight: 150-155

Off season weight: 185-190

What made you decide to compete?

I've always been in awe of muscle and strength. I would watch Mr. Olympia on ESPN when I was little. Helped that I had a huge crush on "AHHNOLD" when I was little.

In preparation for your first show, how long did you train for? If you have competed since, has the time required to prep changed at all? If so, how?

My first show I dieted for 15 wks. Not sure why at the time I chose 15, but it seemed pretty good for a first-timer. I had been training seriously for it for about 15 months. I've competed many times since my first show, and every prep has changed, this will be contradicting, but things have become harder and easier in the same sense. You know what to expect of yourself, but the level of my competition has made preps become more difficult and more serious about how much you improve from one show to the next.

How did you choose a trainer?

I cannot answer because I have always trained myself, and done my own nutrition. This past year, I had what I would call a sound-board. I would contact him for feedback on how I looked, but at the end of the day, I still always decided what I was going to do. He did however, help me load and manipulate water, but that is the just of it.

What do you think is an important, or the most important, thing to consider when trying to find a trainer?

Trust them more than you trust yourself, or at least to the same degree. I know many trainers have done this longer than I have, but I guarantee you they do not know my body, as well as I do, especially with the years of knowledge and trial and error I've already under-gone. I have to have high expectations and respect for them. I want someone that listens and negotiates the best moves/routes to take with me, not be cookie cutter.

I mention in the book that I consider this sport to be kind of a 'selfish' sport. I've given my point of view on this subject. Do you agree? If so, can you

explain how leading a competition prep life interferes with "normal" life? How did you cope with that? What is best piece of advice you can give to competitors regarding this aspect?

I believe this sport is very selfish---It's all about you, and your workouts, your cardio, your food. I feel it's very tough for those that have families to do this sport unless all are very supportive and understand that things are on a "must do" basis in order to bring a good package to the stage. There are many that can balance the lifestyle, but others just getting into the sport, this will take some time management and accurate planning. Since I just have to worry about myself, the only things that I run into are a normal social life; for example being 25 and not wanting to party all the time with friends my age. Even dating--- this can be a nightmare since I choose to do bodybuilding. Most men or mainstream society do not accept or find muscle attractive on a female, let alone one that is trying to always put on size and mature the muscle they do have. It weeds a lot of people in and out of your life, but then you find your true friends and family. Best piece of advice for competitors, and this is in general--- DO YOUR RESEARCH PEOPLE… talk to more than one person about their competition lifestyle and how it has either put a damper in their' lifestyle, or has kinked one's schedule. I feel that I have a fairly good balance, with what I want---but in someone else's eyes, they may want more, you just figure out what you're willing to sacrifice.

I've also stated that this sport is not cheap! Would you please give an estimate of cost for each of the following:

Trainer: I've always trained myself because I have the foundation to. However, I may have an elite trainer this upcoming year which can cost anywhere between $1000-$5000. Depends on how good that person is. Another point to look at is if this person is just training you with the workout aspect or if they are also your nutritional guidance. So the cost above is what I estimated for an ALL-AROUND coach that does both, or at least has feedback for both.

Weekly grocery bill: I average $250-325 a week.

Posing: Again, have always done myself, but a cost for this could range anywhere from $35 a session to $200 for the whole prep, just depends on who you have guiding you.

Tanning: I always do not want to deal with it myself so I will pay the $100-$175 for someone to spray me.

Other than that, I don't normally worry about the tanning bed aspect… I absorb color way too easily to have to fake bake.

Nails: I never get mine done, I am fortunate to have nails that grow long and are durable, so I paint them myself. Others would probably spend about $50-$85

Hair: Normally $100-$150. It is usually packaged with Make-up

Makeup: $80-$150, again is normally package with hair

Suit: This varies per division; I have to have a blank suit which is roughly $150. Then to be more glamorous, I need an evening suit which can range from $200-$1000. This again depends on who you buy from, if it's a rental, or if you try to be cost-efficient and stone a blank one yourself. I've done all of the above, I like all options, especially when the budget changes for me yearly.

Shoes: Most division shoes cost $45-$70… I am no longer wearing heels on stage.

Entry fees (include organizational membership fees): NPC has a running fee of $100 just to compete in NPC/IFBB shows; this has changed every year since I started competing… and when I say change, I mean they've increased the price every year. On top of this fee are sanction/entry fees for the shows in which you choose to compete. Most state/regional shows cost $45-$90; this will depend on the promoter of the show and if the show is popular and very well ran. National shows are more expensive and run $100-$250 now. These prices have increased every year as well since I began competing in 2007.

Anything I missed:

What surprised you the most going through your first preparation? Honestly nothing except for HOW FAST I dropped weight. I was 19 going on 20, and my metabolism was obviously off the charts then.

What was the most difficult part?

Everyone continuously asking, "Oh come on, you can have one little bite can't you?" Or just family gatherings in general or social events and people trying to cram food down your throat.

What do you wish you had known prior to comp and during comp prep?

Honestly nothing, I feel like I had a good base foundation of what I needed to know, I did everything for myself, at the time I had known to competitors that would watch me pose and they would check - in on me and see how I felt through the process, but other than that—the one thing that scared me was being back stage by myself, and not knowing about bikini bite and another competitor having to glue me down, and I was afraid to talk to anyone.

Let's talk about the dreaded "after the competition." I've seen girls never really recover from the "post comp blues." Did you go through this? How did you cope? Any words of advice to help other girls prepare for the physical/mental changes they will experience "after" the show?

N/A

Just for fun:

What food did you miss most during your competition prep?

Sushi and pancakes

What was the first thing you ate after the show?

Sushi or IHOP

What was your favorite competition prep meal?

ALWAYS ALWAYS my oats and protein

Best part of competing?

Always overcoming when you feel like you have

mentally broken down and given it your all; you dig within yourself and continue to keep pushing through to bring a better package each time.

Worst part of competing?

The highs and lows of emotions----sometimes confident, other times you're not sure if you're worthy enough to be one of the elite, (this is especially me speaking from the last two years, not so much previous)

Any final advice for potential competitors?

Do this for you, and about improving you--- being proud of executing diets and workouts that most wouldn't last through in a weeks' time. But always be prepared, always try to learn, and remember to always have fun.

Thank you for your time and feedback!!!

Name: Angela Pearson

Division you compete in: Women's Bodybuilding

Organization(s) you compete in: NPC baby!

Number of years competed: 5

Competition weight: 145-155

Off season weight: 175-180

What made you decide to compete?

I was a competitive cyclist and wanted to improve my pedal stroke. The trainer asked me if I considered competing. I was hesitant at first but I did and my first show was in figure, but the judges said I had legs of a WBB. I waited 2 years to add size to my upper body and competed in bodybuilding in 2010.

In preparation for your first show, how long did you train for?

I can't remember how long I prepped for, for my figure show, but my first bodybuilding show I prepped for 18 weeks.

If you have competed since, has the time required to prep changed at all?

Depending on how fat I get in the off season I can prep up to 24 weeks. That also depends on how many shows I plan on doing.

If so, how?

The last show I did in 2012 I started my prep Jan 1 and

competed July 28th.

How did you choose a trainer?

I chose the trainer/coach I have now based on his track record. I have been with him since 2006. Now he pretty much just does my diet and monitors my physique via pictures.

What do you think is an important, or the most important, thing to consider when trying to find a trainer?

Respect, do you respect this person enough to listen to them and do they respect you enough to be more than a trainer.

I mention in the book that I consider this sport to be kind of a 'selfish' sport. I've given my point of view on this subject. Do you agree?

Yes and no. I believe this sport is self-centered, but it has to be considering that you stand alone on stage to be judged. No because so many people look to us as inspiration and motivation. If we just take the time to explain why we do it, how we do it and that it is like any other extreme no pay sport, others will learn to love it as well or want to live a healthier life.

If so, can you explain how leading a competition prep life interferes with "normal" life?

In the beginning it didn't interfere but caused me to

limit some extra curricula activities, like partying and staying up late. I had to become more organized and spend a little more time preparing my meals for the week.

How did you cope with that?

I knew I had a goal in mind and I did the best I could.

What is best piece of advice you can give to competitors regarding this aspect?

Make sure your support system is in place and understands what it is that you are doing.

I've also stated that this sport is not cheap! Would you please give an estimate of cost for each of the following:

Trainer: During a 24 week contest prep 1500.00

Weekly grocery bill: $125

Posing: $250

Tanning: $100

Nails: Free, I am a nail tech but I charge $80 for hands and feet

Hair: $60

Makeup: $50

Suit: $100-300

Shoes: I don't wear shoes

Entry fees (include organizational membership fees): NPC card = $100, Entry fees $100-200 a show

Anything I missed: Photo shoots can be free, paid for various websites or cost up to $200.

What surprised you the most going through your first preparation? The way my body changed during the final stages. It was like it was full speed ahead towards the end. I was also surprised at how stubborn my body was and how much in the beginning it is more of a trial and error kind of process.

What was the most difficult part?

The most difficult was eating. I was not use to eating so much food. Not at one time but throughout the day. We are conditioned to eat 3 times a day. Changing that to 6 times and although they appeared smaller, they were enough to last til the next 3. Then there were those times that I would eat and be immediately hungry. So managing my meals and water intake was a chore by itself.

What do you wish you had known prior to comp and during comp prep?

Honestly, nothing. If I would have known then what I know now; I probably would not have done it. The entire learning process is what intrigued me. I kept going just to see what would happen. The small changes were the most entertaining from day to day, like, "Oooo that line was not there yesterday." Or,

"OMG I have veins in my abs, really!!!"

Let's talk about the dreaded "after the competition." I've seen girls never really recover from the "post comp blues." Did you go through this? How did you cope?

No. I did everything in reverse.

Any words of advice to help other girls prepare for the physical/mental changes they will experience "after" the show? DON'T OVEREAT BECAUSE YOU THINK YOU CAN. Our bodies take 16-20 weeks to get on stage, but in 20 hours you CAN put on 15lbs!!!

Just for fun:

What food did you miss most during your competition prep?

PIZZA!!!!

What was the first thing you ate after the show?

PIZZA!!!!

What was your favorite competition prep meal?

Eggs, I love eggs. I joke that I can eat eggs with tree bark and be ok!

Best part of competing?

Photo-shoots. I love the camera. Meeting people who enjoy what you do. Even those who just follow the sport.

Worst part of competing?

Insults from people who think you are doing too much and hate the way you look; like being called a man just because they can't do it. Also the creeps that make strange request but there are those who honor them. I am just not one of the ladies that do.

Any final advice for potential competitors?

COUNT YOUR COST BEFORE YOU START! DO YOUR RESEARCH! DO NOT GET ON STAGE UNLESS YOU LOOK THE PART! HAVEFUN!

Thank you for your time and feedback!!!

Thank you!

Name: Holly Renee Iglehart

Division you compete in: Bikini

Organization(s) you compete in: IFPA (Professional division), NPC, WBFF

Number of years competed: 2

Competition weight: 115-122

Off season weight: 125-128

What made you decide to compete?

I was a college track athlete so naturally was in very good shape. When I started nursing school and was no longer competing in college track I gained a little bit of extra weight. I wanted to find something to motivate me to push myself farther than before and continue living a healthy lifestyle. I found a show online and it forced me to stay in the gym and eat clean.

In preparation for your first show, how long did you train for? If you have competed since, has the time required to prep changed at all? If so, how?

I started losing weight in January, but didn't sign up for a show until March. So I would say I dieted/ trained for 8 weeks, but in total I took 4 months to lose 20 pounds. Now I start dieting and increasing training 4-6 weeks out.

How did you choose a trainer?

My first show I did most of the prep on my own, but used a trainer for a few workouts to try out something different towards show time. As far as selecting a trainer, I look at their qualifications- (degree & certifications), as well as their client successes. I also take a look at their philosophy behind training and diet because I want to make sure that their philosophy is similar to my own.

What do you think is an important, or the most important, thing to consider when trying to find a trainer?

I would say knowing what their philosophy is before starting to train with them is the most important thing. If you are a natural athlete, and they are wanting you to take diuretics or cutting agents then you are either wasting your time/ money or you are going to end up doing something against your morals- or vice versa. Know their standpoint before you start!

I mention in the book that I consider this sport to be kind of a 'selfish' sport. I've given my point of view on this subject. Do you agree? If so, can you explain how leading a competition prep life interferes with "normal" life? How did you cope

with that? What is best piece of advice you can give to competitors regarding this aspect?

I believe it is a selfish sport to an extent. I think that you do have to train more than the average person and obviously the diet is way more extreme than most. But I have found that I have been able to continue to my normal activities with little interference. I still go on dates with my boyfriend to the movies, but instead of getting popcorn, I bring my own almonds. When we go to dinner, I order a plain grilled chicken or fish with asparagus without oil. It's possible to still have fun and be training for a show, it's a matter of letting yourself do so. I never stress out about going to long without eating- knowing that I will just double up at my next meal if this happens. Yes- I don't want to go longer than 2-3 hours without eating, but life happens and sometimes you leave the house and forget your chicken breast. My best piece of advice is to not let the prep consume you. If you aren't enjoying what you're doing and still a happy person- then you have lost sight of what competing is all about. Being on stage is only a fraction of the whole process. It is important to enjoy the ride along the way.

I've also stated that this sport is not cheap! Would

you please give an estimate of cost for each of the following:

Trainer: (I no longer utilize a trainer since my boyfriend is a professional bodybuilder and can help with my prep but when I did have a trainer it was approx. $400 for 8 weeks)

Weekly grocery bill: $100-150

Posing: I do all of my own posing training, but a WBFF posing camp costs approximately $100 for a four hour camp.

Nails: $30 manicure/ $30 pedicure

Hair: Stage hair with touchups $45-65

Makeup: Stage make up with touchups $45-65

Suit: My last suit cost $160

Shoes: $200 (my shoes are designer- but I have worn them in 5 shows) plain shoes are around $50

Entry fees (include organizational membership fees): WBFF: Annual membership $175, 1st class entry: $109+ tax= $309 Additional classes entered $75 NPC: Annual membership $100 1st class entry: $50-70= $150-170, IFPA: Annual Membership: $80, entry fee $120, polygraph $40= $240

Anything I missed:

What surprised you the most going through your first preparation?

My first prep I did low carbs, and I would become very forgetful and was also very cranky. After going through that once, I never did low carbs again and I noticed that I was not forgetful and didn't experience any mood swings like I had before.

What was the most difficult part?

The most difficult part is eating the same types of foods over and over again. There are only so many lean meats to choose from and chicken and fish get pretty old after several weeks.

What do you wish you had known prior to comp and during comp prep?

I wish that I would have known that there is such a thing as cutting your calories too low. My first prep I would be eating around 1,000 calories a day and I ended up holding onto fat because my body thought it was starving. Now when I am doing my prep I never go under 1,400 calories a day.

Let's talk about the dreaded "after the competition." I've seen girls never really recover from the "post comp blues." Did you go through this? How did you cope? Any words of advice to

help other girls prepare for the physical/mental changes they will experience "after" the show?

I have gone through this once, and it was caused by my placing. It is so disappointing to work so hard and not place where you feel that you deserve. What helped me is realizing that I didn't do this for anyone else but myself so as long as I felt good about how I looked my placing or what anyone else thought does not really matter.

Just for fun:

What food did you miss most during your competition prep? Doughnuts

What was the first thing you ate after the show?

Cheeseburger and doughnuts (Krispy Kreme)

What was your favorite competition prep meal?

Tilapia and grilled asparagus

Best part of competing?

Walking across the stage

Worst part of competing?

CRAVINGS!

Any final advice for potential competitors?

If you are trying to decide whether to compete or not,

find a show a few months away and sign yourself up! & then there is no turning back.

Main difference between WBFF:

The WBFF is more about the show experience. It is a major production and their goal is to put on a fun and entertaining show for the audience. The venues are extravagant and the music and lighting are over the top. It is a fun, exciting atmosphere, but the actual judging is more along the same structure as a beauty pageant. The judges select the winners based off who they personally like and who they feel will represent the WBFF the best. The NPC/ NANBF/ IFPA have judging criteria and will rank the competitors in order of placing based on who best meets the criteria. In NPC/NANBF/ IFPA you can get feedback from the judges by getting comment cards so that you know what to work on and what you are doing well. It is very helpful as a competitor to know what to improve on for the next show.

Thank you for your time and feedback!

Name: Monique Waters, LMT

Division you compete in: Figure

Organization(s) you compete in: NANBF, soon to be NPC

Number of years competed: First year

Competition weight: 124 lbs

Off season weight: 133 lbs

What made you decide to compete?

I happened to meet a bodybuilder and he had showed me photos of girls because he thought I should compete. I agreed that it would be a good idea and something new for me to try to see what I was made of.

In preparation for your first show, how long did you train for? If you have competed since, has the time required to prep changed at all? If so, how?

I trained about 17 weeks for the first show. I am currently training for a show. I maintained pretty close to contest prep because I didn't want to work that hard all over again so time has been cut down to about 9 weeks since that is when the next show is.

How did you choose a trainer?

Like I mentioned earlier, I happened to meet a bodybuilder and kind of fell into it.

What do you think is an important, or the most important, thing to consider when trying to find a trainer?

You have to find someone who can support you and push you. The thing I loved about my trainer was he could push me and he knew how far he could take me. He took time to spend time with me and speak to me even when we were not in the process of training. I had trouble going back to a somewhat normal diet after the show because I was terrified of gaining a pound and he talked me through that process and got me back on track. You also have to be very comfortable with them, especially if using a man. You basically strip down for these people to a competition suit (which is tiny) so they can critique your physique and watch you pose. At first, I wasn't sure about that, but he made it very clear that I wouldn't have the nerve to get on stage if I had trouble just doing these things in front of him, which made perfect sense.

I mention in the book that I consider this sport to be kind of a 'selfish' sport. I've given my point of view on this subject. Do you agree? If so, can you

explain how leading a competition prep life interferes with "normal" life? How did you cope with that? What is best piece of advice you can give to competitors regarding this aspect?

I agree that it is very selfish. I actually quit dating someone because they felt I spent more time at the gym than with them. This sport is a lifestyle, from the things you eat, to who you hang with, to your schedule, to your attitude. You can't engage in the same activities as your friends or party all night. You can't eat what your family eats. You can't miss workouts. You tend to workout alone unless you have a competition prep buddy or trainer because these are not your average workouts. The sport is expensive so you find yourself setting aside money to pay for food, supplements, trainers, posing, suits, hair, and makeup which takes away from other things you would normally do. Your whole world starts to revolve around your diet and your body. The people around you have to be understanding and support you. Unfortunately, there are many who will not. So either you choose them or this. I choose to have people in my life who have supported my decision to compete and I feel I have made the right decision. It has turned me into a brand new person and I ABSOLUTELY LOVE THE NEW

ME!!

I've also stated that this sport is not cheap! Would you please give an estimate of cost for each of the following:

Trainer: $45 to $60 per session depending on if you buy packages. I used him once a week typically.

Weekly grocery bill: $60 to $70 weekly or around $250 to $300 per month for only myself.

Posing: $40 per session. I would pose once or twice per week for at least 8 weeks.

Tanning: I used the competition spray tanners. It runs about $150 for spray and touch ups throughout show day.

Nails: $27

Hair: $100

Makeup: $100

Suit: $400

Shoes: $50

Entry fees (include organizational membership fees): $150

Anything I missed:

Supplements cost me about $80 per month depending

on how fast I went through them. I also traveled to my show so I paid gas and hotel fees. This was about an additional $400 or so.

What surprised you the most going through your first preparation?

The difference in competition shape compared to just being in shape. These are two completely different things. It took an extreme amount of dedication to get to such a low body fat percentage, but I was also amazed at how well my body took to it. It was a quick process being that I followed all the rules and kept up with the diet and workouts. You can change your body so drastically in a matter of 12 weeks if you follow the program. I lost 30 lbs for my first show. I will be sure to stay close to competition weight from here on out. It is just easier so I am maintaining about 9 lbs from contest weight.

What was the most difficult part?

Most would say dieting and believe me, it is hard, but I was a pretty clean eater already so it was not too bad for me. It was staying away from family functions and friends to avoid temptation and trying to find time to always get in workouts and prep my food. I have a day job, I own a massage therapy business, and I have family. Juggling all that with competition prep was very hard.

What do you wish you had known prior to comp and during comp prep?

I wish I had understood that there is a mental change. I am a very strong woman, but like I said, this is a lifestyle and your views change. I think I gained a very unrealistic view of a woman's body and it was hard to get back to normal and understand that I was the one with an idealistic body image. I would look at girls in shape and I'd think they were a mess because I would look at myself at 10% body fat and wonder why they didn't look like me. I also was so used to being on such a strict schedule and diet, that it didn't just stop the night after the show. I was absolutely terrified to put weight back on. Especially since I was very vocal about my prep and posted Facebook pictures and the whole nine because I knew this would help me promote health and wellness for my business. I felt like everyone was counting on me to always be in competition shape. I did come out of this stage, but it took a few weeks for me to feel normal again and realize that it was ok to put on a few pounds.

Let's talk about the dreaded "after the

competition." I've seen girls never really recover from the "post comp blues." Did you go through this? How did you cope? Any words of advice to help other girls prepare for the physical/mental changes they will experience "after" the show?

I just spoke of this above. I think preparing yourself ahead of time is important. Nobody told me about this. I learned by experience. Luckily my trainer stepped in and helped me through it. I thought it helped to speak to someone and also I was vocal on Facebook and to all of my supporters about how I was feeling and that it was not normal to be in that kind of shape long term and people were very supportive of me. I also made a commitment to continue to eat clean and workout on the regular so I didn't have the fear of putting a major amount of weight back on. I have been able to maintain about 9 lbs. from contest weight without starving and without being at the gym for hours every day. You just have to find your balance. Make a commitment to be healthy. Don't give up on clean eating and working out altogether just because you aren't preparing for a show.

Just for fun:

What food did you miss most during your

competition prep?

SWEET TEA VODKA AND CHUGGING IT AT THE LAKE ON THE BOAT!! Lol, not really a food huh?

What was the first thing you ate after the show?

Ha-ha, well for meal one, I had two soft pretzels, a long island, a shot of tequila, 12 wings, and potato wedges. The next meal was more wings, mashed potatoes and gravy, macaroni and cheese, and the biggest slice of caramel cake I have ever had in my life! It was delicious!

What was your favorite competition prep meal?

Oatmeal. You never realize how much you love oats until someone takes them from you because it is not a carb up day.

Best part of competing?

Realizing how strong you really are, mentally and physically. It is crazy how you change as a person. It was also great meeting other women who were into the sport because everyone is motivated just like you. You learn so much and get so much amazing inspiration. You become an inspiration to others.

Worst part of competing?

Getting your butt to the gym on the days when you

have absolutely no motivation to do so.

Any final advice for potential competitors?

Believe in yourself!! Have fun!! So many people will question why you want this. It is very personal and changes you inside and out for the better. Hold on to that your whole prep or they will discourage you.

Thank you for your time and feedback!!!

Massage Amani

816-210-2934

www.massageamani.massagetherapy.com

Kansas City, MO

Name: Sarah Skinner

Division you compete in: Women's Figure and Physique

Organization(s) you compete in: NPC

Number of years competed: First year.

Competition weight: 135

Off season weight: This will be my first real "off season."(Although I like to call it "preseason.") I'm aiming to staying around 150lbs.

What made you decide to compete?

I love competition, I love working out. I spent a lot of time in the gym and kept getting asked if I was going to compete and always answered , "No, I just want to be strong". Then my boyfriend decided to do a show, so I made the commitment as well. It was the best decision I have ever made.

In preparation for your first show, how long did you train for? If you have competed since, has the time required to prep changed at all? If so, how?

This was my first year competing and I was in 3 shows. All together I trained for my shows for 7 months.

How did you choose a trainer?

John Gorman of Team Gorman was my boyfriend's trainer and I loved his work and the result my boyfriend was seeing. I went with him to a Team Gorman get together and fell in love with the team. They are the greatest most supportive and encouraging group of people I have ever met and it's an honor to be a part of TG.

What do you think is an important, or the most important, thing to consider when trying to find a trainer?

Results. Do your research. Find out how their previous clients have placed and finished, if you like their look. Make sure your trainer is somebody you can really get along with because they become your new best friend. Also be able to trust them, a lot of what you bring to stage is in their hands.

I mention in the book that I consider this sport to be kind of a 'selfish' sport. I've given my point of view on this subject. Do you agree? If so, can you explain how leading a competition prep life interferes with "normal" life? How did you cope with that? What is best piece of advice you can give to competitors regarding this aspect?

This is such a huge question that we "competitors"

could probably all write novels on. It is definitely a selfish sport. It takes time away from family and friends and they won't understand why. It takes time away from a relationship unless you are doing it together. However, the diet of course affects your mood which affects everything!! It's rough very rough however it's also very rewarding and that outweighs the struggles. My advice is don't listen to others when they are upset with you because you aren't going out with them, don't listen to the people that try to say you are unhealthy or look gross and definitely don't listen to the people that try to get you to cheat (1 piece won't kill you). Because the more they see you progress the more interested they get. All of the sudden they start asking you questions about your diet or how to work out etc. Then they start encouraging you and become your biggest fan and then they start implementing it in their own lives. Before you know you could help change somebody's life just by sticking to your guns and staying on track, that part is just as rewarding as being on stage to me. In the end IT'S ALL WORTH IT.

I've also stated that this sport is not cheap! Would you please give an estimate of cost for each of the following:

Trainer: $600-$800 (depending on length of prep)

Weekly grocery bill: outrageous. $100 (Just a guess really. Give or take depending on when I run out of things)

Posing: Came with my trainer, but normally at least $30 for 30 min session. (Minimum)

Tanning: $50 a month then $90 for contest tan

Nails: $80

Hair: I did my own hair but at my first show the price was $70

Makeup:$60

Suit: total $300 and that's cheap!!

Shoes: $65

Entry fees (include organizational membership fees): Wbff - $320 Mayhem- $220, Missouri - $100

Anything I missed:

I spent another $100 on jewelry. Hotel rooms plus gas for both WBFF and Mayhem. If you want stage photos, photo shoots or DVDs that could be another couple hundred dollars or more.

What surprised you the most going through your first preparation? The transformation I made. It was

even more than I thought I was capable of doing!
Never underestimate yourself.

What was the most difficult part?

Missing out on family dinners.

**What do you wish you had known prior to comp
and during comp prep?**

I would have to say, I wish I had known just how
expensive it is. Otherwise everything else was just
such a fun learning experience.

**Let's talk about the dreaded "after the
competition." I've seen girls never really recover
from the "post comp blues." Did you go through
this? How did you cope? Any words of advice to
help other girls prepare for the physical/mental
changes they will experience "after" the show?**

Don't binge- eat after. Take one day to enjoy yourself
then get back to some kind of clean eating so that your
body doesn't rebound horribly. Also this was something
that I actually tried to mentally prepare myself for my
whole prep as well, knowing I would put on weight and
fat, this way I wasn't so distraught over it.

Just for fun:

What food did you miss most during your

competition prep?

Mexican and Dairy Queen

What was the first thing you ate after the show?

Waffle House

What was your favorite competition prep meal?

I love oatmeal and protein powder with cinnamon and Splenda. FYI Walden Farms is a life saver during prep.

Best part of competing?

All of it. I can't one single aspect. I love backstage, I love onstage, I love the wonderful women I get to meet. Every single second of that one day makes the whole prep whether 12 weeks or 34 weeks SO worth it.

Worst part of competing?

If we talking about actual day of show, I would say being so thirsty!!!

Any final advice for potential competitors?

Stick to it, don't give up. Always keep a picture of what you want in your head. I'm going to quote my idol, DLB, "Never Settle. Work, Hustle, Kill." The second you step on stage it will all be worth it.

Thank you for your time and feedback!!!

Name: Kristina Marie Gerhardt

Division you compete in: NPC Women's Physique

Organization(s) you compete in: National Physique Commission

Number of years competed: going on 2

Competition weight: 125 lbs

Off season weight: 135-140

What made you decide to compete?

I have been in the fitness industry for 3 decades. People had always asked me if I competed. I had always dreamed of competing but never took peoples' comments too seriously. Currently I'm in business for myself. my company name is Temple Training and I'm a Personal Trainer , Corrective Exercise and Nutrition Specialist at West County Health and Fitness. It is a serious gym for serious results (on any level). There is so much tenure under one roof how can I not pursue and develop what has been a life-long dream.

In preparation for your first show, how long did you train for? If you have competed since, has the time required to prep changed at all? If so, how?

My first show was the 2011 NPC Midwest Championships in St. Louis. I started dieting about 20 weeks out. That's a long time but I knew I had a tremendous amount of changes (both nutritionally and in composition). Each competition prep is a little different the more my coach and I tune into my body.

How did you choose a trainer?

Choosing a trainer is a very personal thing. The chemistry has to be just right. I had two extraordinary coaches before I latched onto my current coach Kit Kitson with In Shape Nutrition. I have the utmost respect for the persons I have worked with. Getting the right coach for you is kind of like finding the missing puzzle piece. You can MAKE a piece fit or find the one that is just right.

What do you think is an important, or the most important, thing to consider when trying to find a trainer?

Like I said, it's a personal thing. There has to be that certain something. Your trainer has to 'get" you. You have to be able to call or text and they "get" you. You have to be accountable and so do they. You are responsible to them BUT they are responsible for you too.

I mention in the book that I consider this sport to be kind of a 'selfish' sport. I've given my point of

view on this subject. Do you agree? If so, can you explain how leading a competition prep life interferes with "normal" life? How did you cope with that? What is best piece of advice you can give to competitors regarding this aspect?

My life revolves around fitness. So this sport CAN become as selfish as you allow it to. There has to be a balance as in with any sport. The more one puts into an effort the more result one gets. I am fortunate to work and train at the same facility, so I don't spend a lot of time going to and from locations. I eat differently than most everyone in my house but that's ok too. When it comes to competitions, I'm blessed because my family supports me and is right there in the audience to be my cheering section. My son is 10 yrs. old so he is my biggest supporter. I think if you have a large family or small children this sport can surely occupy a lot of time otherwise spent with them. So I'm on the fence of it being a "selfish" sport.

I've also stated that this sport is not cheap! Would you please give an estimate of cost for each of the following:

Trainer: Varies anywhere from $50/per session or flat fees $1000-1200 per 12 week. I don't divulge my personal expenses because I work with various individuals & we help each other.

Weekly grocery bill: Holy cow!!!!! Can run for women $150 on up depending on supplementation.

Posing: My coaches posing fees are included in the trainer fees. But again it varies $40-70 per session. Some people hold boot camps for competition training (nutrition/suit selection/posing/etc.).

Tanning: Tanning pre-show is usually $100-150 & is well worth it. If you go on stage with a bad, muddy or streaked tan …points off. The companies tan you, glue the suits, and gloss you before stage time. You can opt to do it yourself. It would save 75% of the cost, BUT, why take the chance?

Nails: I keep my nails all the time. But plan to get gels or manicure, and a pedicure $50-100.

Hair: I barter with my hairdresser and good friend for hair treatments. But again for someone good..$100+ & if u get extensions $1000+

Makeup: I will get a makeup artist from now on. They are relatively inexpensive (compared to all the other expenses) & range from $50-100. False eyelashes are a must.

Suit: Every division is dif. Bikini and body building suits are more reasonable $120+ & figure and physique suits are all over the board $150 on up to I've seen suits for $1200! You can order suits and make payments. Renting suits and buying used are other great options.

Shoes: Shoes are not worn in physique (yeah). But posing shoes you can find from $40 + and you can bedazzle it yourself.

Entry fees (include organizational membership fees): NPC annual fee is $100. Every comp is different. The classes run from $70 on up depending on the size and level of comp.

Anything I missed: Expect to travel. So you have car rental if you don't want to use your vehicle, gas, and maintenance. There can be airline expenses, hotel accommodations, taxis, etc.

What surprised you the most going through your first preparation? How much nutrition is the key. We all know that nutrition is 80% of a person's success. In the comp world I think its 90%.

What was the most difficult part?

Not letting this whole sport consume you. I have a son and a job I love dearly, so balance is the key.

What do you wish you had known prior to comp and during comp prep?

The sport has changed tremendously over the years. It is a lot more cosmetic than sport related on the women's side. I feel that the harder a person works should be the answer, not how much money one spends on extensions, Botox, augmentation, etc......

Let's talk about the dreaded "after the competition." I've seen girls never really recover from the "post comp blues." Did you go through this? How did you cope? Any words of advice to help other girls prepare for the physical/mental changes they will experience "after" the show?

Thank God I never went through the blues, but it is very real and can be very debilitating. Just always know you have to be tough as nails on the outside but more so, on the inside. After competition, we see our bodies change back to their softer more feminine look and that's hard for a lot of women. It's important to know that in order to make progress we need a little extra weight on our bodies to gain muscle. The extra body fat will be burned during prep....not to worry.

Just for fun:

What food did you miss most during your competition

prep? Peanut butter (it's good for you but not how I eat it) – peanut butter is my crack!!!!

What was the first thing you ate after the show?

FUDGE!!!!!!! Chocolate peanut butter & Lots of it.

What was your favorite competition prep meal?

My chocolate oatmeal pancakes with strawberries.

Best part of competing?

The camaraderie of all the ladies.

Worst part of competing?

The egos that get inflated.

Any final advice for potential competitors?

Go into it knowing competition should only be one facet of your life AND just because you may win a competition or two, does not mean you will stay on top every time. Count your blessings & never forget those that helped you.

Thank you for your time and feedback!!!

Name: Melody Harris

Division you compete in: Bikini

Organization(s) you compete in: AFPA and NPC

Number of years competed: 1

Competition weight: 110

Off season weight: 112-114

What made you decide to compete?

Wow! Well this is a touchy subject! The first time I went to the gym with my now husband he pointed out a couple and said he wanted us to look like them. Naturally I got mad and acquired a hate for that girl. She looked VERY good. Then I asked another about her and found out she was a bikini competitor and a pretty good one at that. I made it my goal to look as good as her. Didn't know it took so much effort! After a little while I became friends with that girl and developed a love for competing. Safe to say I started for the wrong reasons, but now I love it.

In preparation for your first show, how long did you train for? If you have competed since, has the time required to prep changed at all? If so, how?

I started training in January and my first show was in April, so about three months. It was kind of a last minute decision to compete.

How did you choose a trainer?

The girl I didn't care for told me about them! That was actually our first conversation. I chose them because a lot of people seemed happy with them and their results, but I have since decided it wasn't what was best for me.

What do you think is an important, or the most important, thing to consider when trying to find a trainer?

Finding someone who has competed themselves! Not someone who says they know how to do it but doesn't do it themselves. Anyone can book a photo shoot!

I mention in the book that I consider this sport to be kind of a 'selfish' sport. I've given my point of view on this subject. Do you agree? If so, can you explain how leading a competition prep life interferes with "normal" life? How did you cope with that? What is best piece of advice you can give to competitors regarding this aspect?

This is a VERY selfish sport to me. By going through all the training and being disciplined on what you eat, people who don't compete see you as a dud. Or at least they do in my life. A lot of people who aren't as interested in the sport think it's a waste of time to work out so much and not be able to just go out to eat and over indulge in junk. You have to be selfish. If you care about the outcome you have no choice but to do what's best for your body and mental sanity. Just so we all know, going out to eat with our pre-packed meals while our friends eat friend foods and have dessert is not good for our sanity.

I've also stated that this sport is not cheap! Would you please give an estimate of cost for each of the following:

Trainer: $200ish but that's a hell of a deal!

Weekly grocery bill: oh jeez…probably $200

Posing: $60-$120 depending on who you know that's willing to help **you.**

Tanning: $35 a month plus $100-$130 spray for show.

Nails: $35

Hair: $60

Makeup: $60

Suit: $150

Shoes: $60

Entry: $60-$100 for organization card and $50-$70 per

class.

Anything I missed:

What surprised you the most going through your first preparation? How much work it is! This is not a sport for the weak, especially the weak minded.

What was the most difficult part?

Staying mentally focused and training after being told my family didn't support it knowing how much it means to me.

What do you wish you had known prior to comp and during comp prep?

That it's expensive! It's really something you have to prepare your wallet for because it's hard to half ass it and accomplish anything.

Let's talk about the dreaded "after the competition." I've seen girls never really recover from the "post comp blues." Did you go through this? How did you cope? Any words of advice to help other girls prepare for the physical/mental changes they will experience "after" the show?

After competition for me was like getting a tattoo. After you're done you want more! I instantly wanted to start looking for the next show to do. Now what I actually did was over indulge! Right after my show I managed to get myself in a horrible skinny fat condition like I was before the show training. I know this time I'll do it a lot differently. Instead of going off the deep end I'd say hold down the training and stick with your trainer so even in the off season you're making changes for the next show you won't regret near as much.

Just for fun:

What food did you miss most during your competition prep?

CEREAL!

What was the first thing you ate after the show?

Pizza and it didn't even taste good!

What was your favorite competition prep meal?

Chicken! I really like chicken.

Best part of competing?

The rush of show day, the final tan, hair and make-up, the glamorous look, and the chance to size up the competition… finally.

Worst part of competing?

Being the first to go on stage! It was so scary!

Any final advice for potential competitors?

Stop talking about it and do it! It'll show in the end!!

Thank you for your time and feedback!!

Chapter 18

Q & A

Part 3: Professional Photographer

Thank you for taking the time to answer some questions for the readers. Most competitors become interested in scheduling a professional shoot while preparing for a competition in order to capture all their hard work and, obviously, their amazing physique. I know when I booked my first ever photo shoot, which happened to be with you, I was kind of unsure what to expect, what I should take to wear, and exactly how much time to allot. Your feedback, information, and tips will be of tremendous help to those out there who are looking to schedule a photo shoot and don't know what the whole process entails.

How long have you been taking Professional Photos?

I've been shooting Professional, meaning full time for my living, for four years. I've been shooting much longer, sometimes for pay, but not full time. I bought my first camera when I was in 3rd grade.

What occasions are you usually hired to shoot?

I'm usually hired to do personal shoots, but getting more into weddings in 2013. Have also shot parties and get asked to do a lot of lingerie shoots.

I know some of your pictures have been featured in magazines. Which magazine are you most excited about being published in?

I like Planet Muscle magazine. Jeff Everson has been around for years. His ex-wife is Cory Everson. He treats photographers well and right.

Let's say you are shooting a competition and offering private shoots that same weekend, what is the max number of shoot's you will book?

Depends on the contest; if it is large, the judging will go late so I book less. I have done as many as 16 in one weekend.

Where can someone go to find out where/when you will be shooting and book a time slot?

Facebook and my website. www.dougjantzphotography.com

If a competitor books a shoot with you, how much time should they allow?

1-1 ½ hours; although usually about an hour is

sufficient. If I'm not too busy and the shoot is going well, it will probably go longer.

Do you know your locations ahead of time, or do you kind of wing it?

Both! If I'm going to a town that is new, I have to wing it. Location is the most asked question and most of the time the least important. Location matters very little. I've done a shoot on a loading dock behind a restaurant, one photo from it being on the cover of Planet Muscle magazine!

Where is your favorite location to shoot?

I loved Pikes Place in Seattle. But I probably have more fun shooting in Springfield, MO than anywhere so far. I feel more at home there I guess!

How many changes of clothes do you suggest a competitor bring?

3-4. Always better to bring more and not use them than to wish you would have brought something.

I know some photographers are kind of "iffy" on their legitimacy. Any warning signs a girl can look for when choosing a photographer?

Asking for nudes right off! I know guys who do this. Also beware of photographers who do "TF" shots all the time. This means, "Trade for…whatever." If you want really consistently good photos, pay someone. Is he/she known by people you know? References? Published in a "real" magazine, not just online magazines? I flirt LOL, but some guys go so way beyond flirting. Are his comments toward you making you uncomfortable? That is a warning sign. Any professional memberships? I am a member of Nikon Professional Services, meaning Nikon has checked me out and validated me and my work.

What is number one "concern" you hear from competitors?

That he or she isn't in good enough shape for photos, too fat, etc., and the location of the shoots. I hear those two more than anything else. Check out the FAQ page of my website for help on all of these concerns.

What is best piece of advice you can give to someone who is preparing for a photo shoot?

Relax and just prepare for fun! Makeup is a little heavier than normal and be sure to wear eyeliner on top AND bottom. Get your hair done. I have had several show up for shoots with hair just hanging and no makeup on. Don't do it!! Don't be concerned about being in contest shape either. A few more pounds are good!

Do you have a personal website, Facebook page, and/or contact information girls can reach you at to discuss booking a photo shoot?

Facebook (Doug Jantz), email: Doug@dougjantz.com, or website: www.dougjantzphotography.com .

Extra Info:

Besides Fitness, I have shot a lot of lingerie and bikini pictures. If there is something you would like to shoot with me, just ask.

Amanda adding comment:

I asked Doug to provide this information because I have personally used his services twice, and have always been extremely pleased with his mannerism, professionalism, creative eye, and just overall expertise in photography. He has always made the experience extremely fun and relaxing, not to mention the amazing pictures he takes. I HIGHLY recommend his services to anyone who might have access to him. His work can be seen on his Facebook page and website, as well as MY Facebook page (Amanda Larson),and the "About the Author" picture at the end of the book. He is also extremely reasonably priced for the amount of USABLE pictures you receive. I don't think I've ever come out of a shoot with Doug that I didn't have at least 50 or more usable pictures (meaning without eyes being closed, mouth open weird, or something wrong with the picture.)

Thank you for your time and information!

Chapter 19

Q and A

Part 4: Judges

Rebecca Woody

First of all, thank you for taking the time to answer these questions for me. I know that there will be many girls out there who will greatly benefit from your experience and knowledge. I'm sure you know, being a competitor, there is so much to this sport and looking back on your first competition you think, "If only I would have known." So, I appreciate you helping new and future competitors in their journey to the stage.

Let's start by providing some competition background? When did you start competing, in what division, and what achievements did you accomplish?

I've been a NPC Bodybuilding competitor from 1986 to 2001 competing in over 28 competitions in multiple classes consisting of Open, Masters and Couple's. Highest achievement 1st place NPC 1990 National Light weight division and 4th in 1991 at over age 40 competed again at age 53 after 10 years off, took 2nd in Open and Masters.

How long have you been judging?

I've been an NPC judge from 1987 to 1997. Currently judging or Head Judge for the NANBF since 2000.

Can you tell me a little about the organization that you are involved in?

I know that NANBF has been promoting their contest in Kansas City for 17-18 years now. It is another venue for those that choose to compete on a natural stage since they possibly cannot compete on other venues or chose not to. This association became the leader in the drug free movement.

What constitutes a "Natural" show and how is it tested?

A band substance list is posted on websites that promote the 'natural' shows. A polygraph is given prior to the contest. If the competitor wins his/her class, they are required to give a urine sample which is then tested.

Obviously there has been an expansion in the categories in this sport. When I first competed, there was no such thing as "bikini" and now it is

the most popular division it seems. Even as of the last couple years, it divided out even further by adding "Women's Physique." Many girls getting ready to enter a competition aren't quite sure which category would be best for them. Could you please discuss the top 2-3 characteristics of each category? (example: leanness, muscle mass, symmetry)Bikini, Figure, Women's Physique, Bodybuilding, Fitness.

Figure, Women's Physique and Bodybuilding:

SYMMETRY: Does the upper body match the lower body? Front match back? Even in leanness. IS Lower as lean as upper; Upper as lean as lower? X frame.

MUSCULARITY; Looking for muscularity, definition, striations with full muscle bellies. Not flat or looks like a concentration camp competitor, swimmer or marathon runner.

PRESENTATION; how well you perform quarter and mandatories. Fluid movements, suit choice and fits well. Skin tone and color should be even.

Bikini is a softer look, not looking for caps on shoulders, back muscularity or leg development, but we are looking for well tone individual, abs would be a plus, at least leanness in midsection. Suit should flatter that person and skin tone/color should be even. Judges should be forgiving if glutes are softer than per say figure woman.

Fitness judged on flexibility, strength, aerobic ability and dance/rhythm a plus. Athletic Physique and well-toned.

As a judge I'm sure there is a characteristic that you would consider a "must have" and a "must not have" in each category. Obviously a Bodybuilder would not do well in a Bikini division. Will you please put it in simple terms for us on what you consider the MOST important to have and to NOT have in each category?

The ability to separate bodybuilding vs. figure vs. bikini, will admit that judges struggle with this portion and are given a criteria to look for plus briefed by promoters' with each of these classes. My personal opinion is women's bodybuilding, as we know it, is fading. Competitions are not as large as in previous years; even at the USA and National levels have decreased. I look to see women's physique taking its place. With that said, all federations are struggling to judge these new classes that are coming at a fast speed. What judges are looking for is still a painful process that has not yet been completely determined; it's a work in progress. A 'must not have' is a judge favoring muscle in a bikini class!

In your opinion, how much importance do you give to: posing, suit choice, hair, nails, makeup etc? I mean, are the nails and eyelashes really THAT important?

A well- fitting suit for both men and women is the most important. Second posing, so many cannot show their bodies, as a judge if I can't see it, example back or lat spread, how can I judge? You can't present it, I'll give it to the person who can. Makeup is important, stage makeup should be required for women, and they are washed out with the bright lights if they do not wear more than average for the stage vs. day makeup. Lashes are not that important, more than eye shadow, lots of eye shadow and lips, nice to see them with color. Ok, don't care if you manicure your finger nails, but for crying out loud, get a pedicure, nothing like looking at toes hanging from your ill fitted shoes looking like a condor!

Continuing on with the topic of judging, please inform us of how a judge is chosen/trained?

You can be invited or request to test judge. NANBF hands a criteria to follow as a guide line, usually the promoter is willing to answer any and all of your questions before you test, he she prefers you to be a present or past competitor.

Can you explain the whole judging process, scoring, high/low scores etc and how the placements are ultimately decided?

Depending upon the requirements of each federation; NPC favors that you have competed; you are tested by being allowed to sit on a judging panel during the morning show. You are then graded based on the majority of where the judges placed the top 5 competitors in each class. NANBF basically has the same system but favoring all placements of each class no matter how small or large; test judge should expect over a 90% grade is acceptable. Past or present competitor is expected.

Have you ever seen a tie? How is a tie decided?

Symmetry and scoring breaks the tie or the head judge will do this task. It is rare, only had to do this once in a men's overall and I went for the symmetry they all had plenty of muscle.

Do you encourage girls to contact judges after the

show to get feedback?

As a NPC competitor for years, I never had to question a judge or wanted to; always knew what my weaknesses were and strengths. Understanding it is different now and judges make themselves more approachable, which is a plus, so I encouraged positive feedback.

You obviously see many first time competitors. What do you, personally, deem to be the number one "rookie" mistake? Any piece of advice to avoid this?

Physique is not ready, be it not enough muscle or not having a good diet. Then if by chance they have both, they cannot present their fine- tuned body correctly with mandatory poses. I'm an advocate of seeking help, a good trainer, one who understands the sport attempting to undertake. Their ultimate goal is to work themselves out of a job. A rare individual could do without but that is rare for first timers, unless they have been building.

In closing, if you could give one piece of advice to girls reading this, what would it be?

Whatever class you decide to do, after building your frame in the gym, the rest is 90% diet and 10%

training. Keep in mind this is just a sport, very few make a living off of this.

Thank you so much for your time and input!

Kim Seeley

First of all, thank you for taking the time to answer these questions for me. I know that there will be many girls out there who will greatly benefit from your experience and knowledge. I'm sure you know, being a competitor, there is so much to this sport and looking back on your first competition you think, "If only I would have known." So, I appreciate you helping new and future competitors in their journey to the stage.

Let's start by providing some competition background? When did you start competing, in what division, and what achievements did you accomplish?

I actually started lifting for real in 1996 but didn't actually compete until 1999. Funny thing; when I got going, there was no such thing as figure, let alone bikini or any of the other divisions we have now. Our choices were female body building and fitness, so I chose the actual sport of "fitness". At the time when I developed the competition interest or the "bug" as I call it; I couldn't find a supportive local level circuit for fitness so I did some research & I found a Miss Fitness

USA competition in Chicago which wasn't too far to make the trip. I competed with Ms Fitness USA until 2001. After a lot of soul searching about what I wanted for this new found hobby, I switched federations in late 2001 to the NPC. Have been there ever since!! Eventually earning professional status in fitness and becoming an IFBB pro in 2004.

How long have you been judging?

Shortly after turning pro I became involved on the local level judging. I tested out successfully and have been judging shows in our district ever since. I am part of the NPC team that has Missouri, Arkansas & Kansas. So roughly 8 years!

Can you tell me a little about the organization that you are involved in?

The NPC is the acronym for the National Physique Committee. It is the amateur division paired with the professional division which is the IFBB or the International Federation of Body Building. Lots of acronyms out there aren't there?

The NPC/IFBB is the oldest, most prestigious of any federation on planet earth. We are the drivers/inventors of many of the changes in our sport. The leaders if you will on the developments of figure/physique and so on. However we can't claim the title of developing bikini. We stole that idea from others and boy what a huge change it has created!

I call us the NFL of the bodybuilding world.

I've come across many first time competitors or those who are used to competing in the "Natural" circuit who really want to try a NPC show, but are scared due to the stigma of it being associated with steroids. I try to explain that they should not view it that way, but more of a "Non- tested" organization. What do you think of that association? Do you feel that natural competitors can be just as competitive on a NPC stage?

Ughhh…This is something that drives me absolutely insane.

Why wouldn't a natural competitor be as competitive? So are you, or are other people saying every single person that is in the NPC is using steroids? It's just plain silly, and not truthful.

I will be just blunt I guess, "Either you have the genetic potential or you don't". Period …end of it…..

This is actually what "drives the bus" for the NPC. The federation is so extremely large and our process is so amazing, that it makes no difference one way or the other…meaning if it is tested….or if it is not. You can be on every illegal banned substance under the sun and still can get your ass handed to you in the NPC circuit. I've seen it plenty of time. Drugs are not synonymous with the NPC; nor are they synonymous with winning. I hope I never see a bikini girl on steroids! LOL

I'll use one of my Kim "funnisms" to clarify and make a point…

If you are a genetic mess, with poor bone structure, and are unsymmetrical naturally, no matter how hard you work, nor how many drugs you choose to do… it can ever fix that…this is regardless of how conditioned or how big you become. A turd is still a turd no matter what color frosting! Again, the NPC is the epitome of the genetic ideal. Drugs or not, we house the most amazing athletes ever.

How many times have you attended a natural drug tested event and a "genetic ideal" shows up and wins it all, yet people STILL make rude comments about that individual using things or covering up something? Like it's too good to be true. It's very sad. My attitude when I joined the NPC was who cares? I'm gonna jump in and see where I hang, because I wanted to hang with the best and often the best will be hated on ….no matter what.

Obviously there has been an expansion in the categories in this sport. When I first competed, there was no such thing as "bikini" and now it is the most popular division it seems. Even as of the last couple years, it divided out even further by adding "Women's Physique." Many girls getting ready to enter a competition aren't quite sure which category would be best for them. Could you please discuss the top 2-3 characteristics of each category? (example: leanness, muscle mass, symmetry)Bikini, Figure, Women's Physique, Bodybuilding, Fitness.

Ok, let's first say everyone is" ideal" in the way they are made for each category…bone structure and shape. I would say the best way to sum it up, is that there are degrees of muscularity and leanness within each category.

1. Bodybuilding: The bigger the better…that is if all the parts and pieces go well together in a symmetrical harmonious way. In body building there is no such thing as "too lean". This is the king daddy of our

extreme. The shape is an X. Tiny waist!

2. Figure: lean but not to the conditioning of a body builder, has some muscle that is clearly definable to the eye... but again not near to the degree of a body builder. The shape is more of a Y or a martini glass. This doesn't mean that figure girls don't have legs... they do...it's just that the legs are not equal to that of the upper body proportions. Glutes have some roundness and fullness to them. Tiny waist & full round delts are a must. Lats must be wider than the tushy for sure.

3. Physique: this is big figure...not body building. It's for our figure girls who carry more muscle without even trying. The conditioning once again, is still that of a figure girl. They just get to display it with an artistic routine similar to the way bodybuilders do, so this is a big Y shape! All the same must-haves apply!

4. Bikini- this category is still in the works. The degree of muscularity is far less than figure, but yes they still must have some. The shape is more

hour glass like and there should be no extreme look to the muscle groups. Athletic looking and lean. (Yes I did say lean). Often just as lean as a figure athlete but since they don't hold as much muscle; its appearance is totally different. Tiny waist is once again and always the thing to possess with physique sports.

As a judge I'm sure there is a characteristic that you would consider a "must have" and a "must not have" in each category. Obviously a Bodybuilder would not do well in a Bikini division. Will you please put it in simple terms for us on what you consider the MOST important to have and to NOT have in each category?

I think if you refer to the last question it might sum it up. The degree of muscle and the degree of conditioning all play a roll. I'm going to sound like a record, but for all these divisions it's all about the bone structure and how the muscle sits upon it.

Kim, I admittedly don't know much about the "Fitness" category. You being an IFBB Pro-Fitness competitor I'm relying on you discuss this category. Just from the shows I have personally competed in, it seems that this category is kind of

disappearing. What do you think has caused this? Any overall thoughts about the Fitness category?

I love Fitness and believe it's the most athletic division in the whole NPC. It takes tons of athletic ability as well as the ability to get as lean as a figure competitor.

Figure didn't even exist as an option when I began competing. When it was introduced as a division in 2000, that basically put the nail in the Fitness "coffin," then when Bikini came along, it sealed it. It is safe to say that Figure changed Fitness forever.

You and I have discussed in great length the whole judging process as far as the winner might not be the "ideal" yet they still win. I know I've seen competitions where I was confused as to how the final placements were decided, therefore contacted you regarding it. Your explanation regarding "who sucks the least" cleared it up a TON for me. Will you explain it to those reading?

It's true! Judges are not finders of great physiques, we are finders of flaws, and we do that on purpose. In fact, we usually only give feedback on what needs to be worked on. So, basically judging comes down to whoever has the least amount of flaws (and we all have them by the way). The competitor with the least amount of flaws is the winner. You must remember, it's about EVERYTHING flowing together; front matches back and top matches bottom. It's not just about muscle or who is the biggest; body fat is just as important.

Another concept you helped me with was picturing the "X" vs the "martini glass." Can you discuss?

X: This is basically for bodybuilding. This means that the development of the legs is equal to the development of the upper body, separated by a tiny waist. The overall look is that of an "X."

Y: This is the characteristic for Figure and Women's Physique. The upper body development is bigger than the leg development, although you must still have adequate leg muscle. The legs must not compete with the upper body and the sweep on the quad should not over power the width of the back. Basically you cannot be quad dominant.

In your opinion, how much importance do you give to: posing, suit choice, hair, nails, makeup etc? I mean, are the nails and eyelashes really THAT important?

First and foremost; it is in fact a physique contest. This above everything else is the main thing that is judged, especially at an amateur level show. We won't penalize a girl on the local level for posing poorly or having terrible make up skills… however; she certainly will be TOLD about it if she chooses to ask the judges for feedback. At the national level, these things are crucial because the bodies are typically on more of an even playing field. The little things will begin to separate out those who are truly equal when it comes to the actual side by side comparisons.

To answer your question: for me? Very important…..Posing poorly and the suit cut being wrong are the biggest mistake athletes make. If you pose incorrectly it will not show the development you have. (or hide what you don't) Athletes who do not open up the lats both on the front and back pose just kill the "width" illusion on stage. Your actual suit cut can make you or break you (if your body is on par). If all things are equal in the physique aspect; even at the local level …without a doubt… posing, presentation, suit selection etc. are going to be scrutinized. It is a show; attention to detail is important.

Again, the local level is a learning stepping stool for athletes. We want to better them for their preparations as they move up to more competitive shows.

Continuing on with the topic of judging, please inform us of how a judge is chosen/trained?

Showing interest is where it begins!

Simply ask your regional chair- person and let he or she know that you're interested. Having an interest in the sport is going to be a common factor. You need to follow the sport and enjoy it on some level. Experience in it will only help.

Once the interest is expressed you will begin the test judge process. You must pass three actual shows testing.

Can you explain the whole judging process, scoring, high/low scores etc. and how the placements are ultimately decided?

Have you ever seen a tie? How is a tie decided?

Many times! The score keeper will go back and look at the two athletes who are tied and go down the column of all the judges' scores to count who has the most high scores between the two. The athlete who had more individual high scores overall will result in the higher placement.

Do you encourage girls to contact judges after the show to get feedback?

YES! Please yes. Without sounding mean, it's just not my job to come find you. Come find us and talk to us. We as NPC judges are here at this level to help you. THAT is our job. But we will not know if you are interested in help or moving on if we don't know about it. You must talk to us! Try to do it right after the show if possible or at least within the week. Many judges move on to a new sea of bodies the following weekend and it becomes a blur if you wait too long.

Tips on this subject:

1.   Talk to us even if you win. Why? The NPC local level is "introductory". Just because you win here does not mean you are ready to move on. You are judged and compared against who shows up in your class. At nationals you will be compared to many other winners all across the US. It becomes a new ball game there!

2.   Talk to all of us! Yes, all of us. The sport by nature has some subjectivity to it. It just does. There is a diverse panel of people with different backgrounds and preferences. While we are to follow the guidelines and all of us do…personal preference will often come out when it comes to feedback time. I truly think the only way to toss out confusing subjectivity is by speaking to each judge and then and only then… using

what the majority of the panel agrees upon.

I.e.: if every judge on the panel says to improve your delts, guess what? That's gospel...improve your delts! All other things that are mixed, just toss out.

You obviously see many first time competitors. What do you, personally, deem to be the number one "rookie" mistake? Any piece of advice to avoid this?

If you choose to compete, and are going to invest this much hard work, then go ahead and INVEST the money to get help!

Hire someone who is professional, not just a pro athlete either but an actual pro at what they do....whether it be the make-up artist, the tanning company, suit maker, nutritionist etc.

Do your homework and find the right team of people to aide in your success. It is a great feeling to walk away knowing full well you left nothing on the table as far as your preparation was concerned.

In closing, if you could give one piece of advice to girls reading this, what would it be?

"Make sure this endeavor is about the journey and not simply the destination."

For many of us, making it to the finish line is a daunting yet exhilarating process. The physical and emotion investment is really quite deep, and once you cross to the end, often times it's the feeling of, "Huh? all that for this?" …meaning the time on stage is brief…even if you win!

I believe for the masses, this unique sport is an amazing hobby. Yes, a hobby. There is a select unique few; who can live off of it and can prosper, but for the rest of us it is something we do and not what we are.

This hobby is an investment in your health; mentally, physically, and often spiritually. It can truly test what we are made of and create special talents that can help in other aspects of life. Commitment, dedication, discipline, perseverance, what better traits to possess?

But at the same time, be mindful that the sport only has one winner rewarded with a trophy at the end of the day…JUST one. You will not always win. In fact it's a rare and amazing thing to win. Enjoy it while it happens, but most of all…ENJOY the journey….not simply the destination. The human spirit wants to win, and in a subjective sport, it won't happen every time so ensure that it happens every day during the process. Measure your success by achieving what your goals were for doing it in the first place. This will ensure we can win on some degree even if it wasn't recognized by a trophy.

Thank you so much for your time and input!

Kim can be contacted via Facebook: Kim Seeley IFBB Pro

About the Author

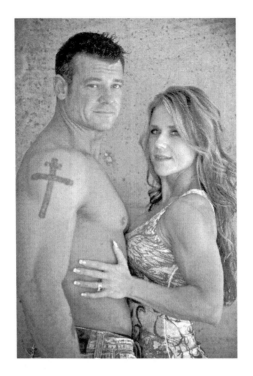

Amanda Larson has been competing since 2005, and earned her Pro Figure status in the WBFF, her first time on stage. Over the years she has successfully competed in the NPC; earning the chance to compete in the National level circuit. In 2012 she switched from Figure to Women's Physique and earned a first place win in her first Physique appearance. A few weeks later she competed in the USA's in Las Vegas and placed 6th in her first National appearance. She continues to train in hopes of earning her Women's Physique IFBB pro card in 2013.

Amanda is married to her husband, Lee, who

competes in the NPC as a super heavy weight bodybuilder. They are both sponsored by Supplement Supersource (http://www.supplementsupersource.com) and offer nutrition and workout plans to people who wish to compete, or just have the desire to get in better shape. They are also both judges for the AFPA (www.kcbodybuildingonline.com) and can be contacted at amandalarson73@gmail.com or found on Facebook: Amanda Larson and/or Lee Larson for questions or pricing packages.

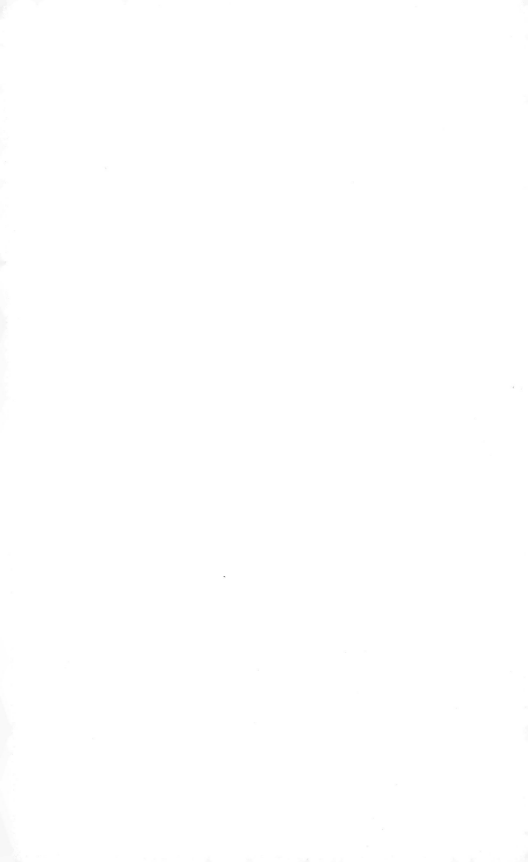

Made in the USA
Lexington, KY
19 February 2013